To better sleep!

Copyright © 2014 by Jeffrey R. Prager DDS, D.ACSDD
All rights reserved. This book or any portion thereof
may not be reproduced or used in any manner whatsoever
without the express written permission of the publisher
except for the use of brief quotations in a book review.

Printed in the United States of America

First Printing, 2014

ISBN 978-0-9915876-0-5

Jeffrey R. Prager DDS, D.ACSDD
The Bellingham Smile Care and Sleep Center
1420 King Street, Suite B, Bellingham, WA 98229
360-671-4552 | info@bellinghamsmiles.com
www.BellinghamSmiles.com

CONFESSIONS
—— OF A ——
RENEGADE DENTIST

Read only at the risk of:
Increasing your confidence, enhancing the quality of
your life, and significantly improving your health.

by Dr. Jeffrey R. Prager

Dedication

No dentist can do what they do alone. I could never make a difference in the lives of my patients without the unflagging support and loyalty of my dedicated and talented team—the finest I have ever assembled. Many thanks and much gratitude to Lisa, Shawn, Jade, Danielle, Stassya, Sarah, and Doris, for their trust, dedication, and willingness to go the extra mile for our valued patients.

Contents

CHAPTER 1: Improve Your Health, Increase Your Confidence, and Enhance the Quality of Your Life — 9

CHAPTER 2: It's All about You. What's Best for the Patient? — 11

CHAPTER 3: Do You Want a Dentist Up-to-Date on the Latest and Most Comfortable Techniques? — 13

CHAPTER 4: I Became a Dentist because of a 12-Year-Old Boy in 1960s San Diego — 15

CHAPTER 5: Does the Thought of Regular Checkups Stress You Out? — 17

CHAPTER 6: Shock Factor—Oral Health Impacts Your Overall Health — 19

CHAPTER 7: The Oral Health/Systemic Disease Connection — 23

CHAPTER 8: "Dental Terror"—a Solution to Reduce or Even Eliminate Your Fear and Anxiety - Introducing NuCalm—Imagine Enjoying Your Dental Appointment! — 25

CHAPTER 9: Gum Disease and Tooth Loss—an Innovative, Smart, and Comfortable Solution — 33

CHAPTER 10: Gum Disease Treatment without Invasive Surgery—LANAP® is Good News — 39

CHAPTER 11: Your Own Teeth Are Your Best Teeth—You Want to Keep Them! — 43

Five Tightly Guarded, Closely Held Secrets…
Secret 1: Why Each Tooth is Critically Important—If You Lose a Tooth, Replace It! — 47
Secret 2: You Don't Know the 60/40 Rule — 49
Secret 3: Dentistry Isn't Expensive but Dental Neglect Is — 51
Secret 4: Only Two Things Cause Tooth Loss—Control 'Em and You'll Keep 'Em — 53
Secret 5: Dental Insurance Is NOT What You Think It Is — 55
Bonus Secret: The Real Truth about "Dental Vacations" — 57

Contents Cont

CHAPTER 12: Does Snoring Drive You or Your Bed Partner Crazy? — 59

CHAPTER 13: Snoring Is a Literal Wake-Up Call—the Message? Something is Wrong — 61

CHAPTER 14: Sleep Apnea Is a Serious Sleep Disorder with Many Potential Health Hazards — 63

CHAPTER 15: How Do You Know If You Have Sleep Apnea? — 67

CHAPTER 16: There Are Only Four Treatments for Sleep Apnea — 69

CHAPTER 17: Sleep Like a Baby, Wake Refreshed, Experience More Energy and Vitality — 75

CHAPTER 18: Chronic Headaches and Migraines Treated by a Dentist? Really? — 77

CHAPTER 19: Drugs Don't Cure Headaches — 83

CHAPTER 20: Real and Lasting Headache Relief — 85

CHAPTER 21: How Our Therapy Process Helps Your Headaches and Migraines — 87

CHAPTER 22: Do You Offer "Regular Dental Services" like Cleaning, Filling Cavities, Crowns and Preventive Work? You Bet! — 91

CHAPTER 23: Easy and Efficient Ways to Keep Your Teeth Clean, Even if You Hate Flossing — 95

CHAPTER 24: I'm Terrified of the "Needle" and of Pain—Help! — 97

CHAPTER 25: I've Never Liked My Smile, What Can I Do?: Cosmetic Dentistry Solutions Improve Your Smile, Enhance Your Looks, and Increase Your Confidence — 101

CHAPTER 26: FACE IT—TFE is the Best Way to Show Off Your Smile — 107

CHAPTER 27: Free Teeth Whitening for Life — 109

CHAPTER 28: Last Word — 111

Foreword

We know that you might hate going to the dentist and despise everything associated with dentistry. You might think all dentists and dental offices are alike and that if you've had a bad experience, you're never going to have a good one.

If you've experienced pain at the dentist, you might think pain and dentistry go hand-in-hand and so you avoid dental treatment like the plague. We get it. This book is designed to bust myths, teach you some fascinating things about your health and help you improve your life in ways that might surprise you.

We'll share lots of great information with you—from our perspective and from our patients' viewpoints as well. I promise, this book is all about you. First, I want to put you at ease by telling you a little about The Bellingham Smile Care and Sleep Center, who we are, and how we came to have our unique philosophy and perspective.

> DISCLAIMER: THIS BOOK IS NOT INTENDED AS MEDICAL ADVICE AND IS FOR INFORMATIONAL PURPOSES ONLY. BEFORE MAKING ANY DECISION REGARDING YOUR HEALTH, PLEASE CONSULT A LICENSED HEALTH CARE PRACTITIONER.

"When you come in for an appointment, Dr. Prager and his staff make you feel cared about as a person, not just as a client. Not only is the customer service exceptional, but they offer technology you just don't find in other dental offices. Dr. Prager is so diversified with his training that he offers more than just dental care. From headaches to sleep issues, this clinic seems to have it all. If I could recommend any dentist in town, it would be Dr. Prager's office—they truly go the extra mile for their clients."

Jackie Griffith – Ferndale, WA

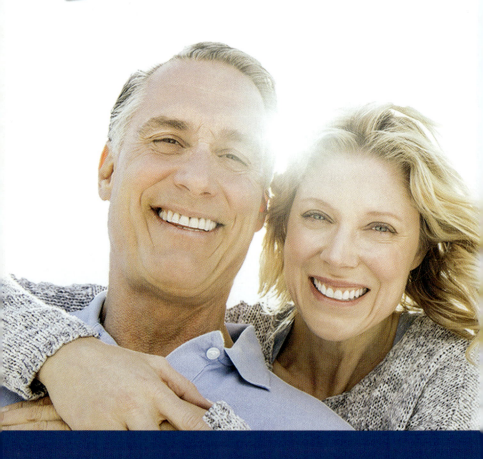

Chapter 1

Improve Your Health, Increase Your Confidence, and Enhance the Quality of Your Life

"You will observe with concern how long a useful truth may be known, and exist, before it is generally received and practiced on." – Benjamin Franklin

At The Bellingham Smile Care and Sleep Center, we offer many solutions for our patients that you may not associate with dentistry. For example, we treat sleep disorders and migraines. We treat snoring and TMJ (jaw joint) problems. We save teeth other dentists give up on. In fact, patients come to us for such diverse treatments that we're often asked if we do "normal" things like fill cavities and clean and repair teeth. The answer is absolutely YES. We do . . . every day!

And our philosophy is a bit different than other dental offices. Our goal is to improve your health, increase your confidence, and enhance the quality of your life. If you're uncertain—even skeptical—about how that can happen through dentistry, then this book is for you. I think you'll find it an informative, eye-opening read and a great reference. Please share it with your friends and family members.

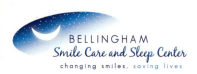
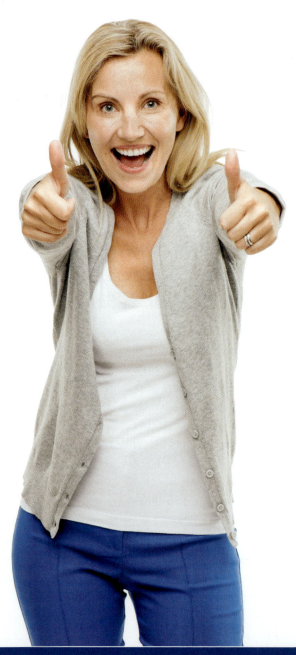

Chapter 2

It's All About You. What's Best for the Patient?

We approach everything we do with this question: What is best for our patients?

That may sound too simple, or even obvious, but I'm discouraged by the way so many of my colleagues do what's best or easiest for them—not their patients. My purpose here isn't to put others down; that's not my style. I do believe, however, that it's important to stand for what we believe in. I thought long and hard about how direct to be in this book and I decided that it was best to stick to what I believe in: doing what's best for my patients—and that includes calling it like I see it and sharing that with you.

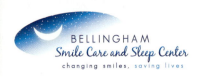

Ever Wonder Why Someone Chooses Dentistry as a Profession?

I'm Dr. Jeffrey Prager and I've been practicing dentistry for 35 years — 28 years here in Bellingham.

Like most careers, dentistry has its share of stress. The profession requires lots of ongoing study and hours of intense concentration. Have you ever noticed how tiring thinking and concentrating is? It still surprises me. Dentists spend a lot of time with patients who are scared to come into the office—that's stressful for us too.

Practicing dentistry requires lots of hours of sitting, bending, and twisting. We make sure the patient is comfortable, but most of us dentists suffer from neck or back problems—or both. Mine were so severe at one point it seemed surgery was the only option. However, I searched out a very successful alternative treatment because I love what I do; giving it up was never an option—I have too many people to help.

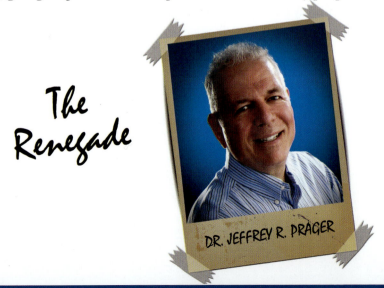

Chapter 3

Do You Want a Dentist Up-to-Date on the Latest and Most Comfortable Techniques?

"He who cures a disease may be the skill-fullest, but he that prevents it is the safest physician."
– Thomas Fuller

I see my career as a dentist like peeling layers of an onion. Every year there are new things to learn and new advances that make what we do easier for patients. I'm totally committed to continuing education because I don't want to miss out on any methods or techniques that could make a difference for even one of my patients.

Some dentists practice the same way year after year—using what they learned years ago in dental school; they don't add or learn new technologies or techniques over their years of practice. That's an entire career where every year is more or less the same; they don't add anything new to their knowledge base or skill set. That would never work for me. I might be nuts, but so far, I've practiced differently each year for 35 years, learning and adding to my skills every year.

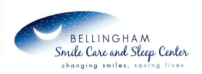

I think you have to keep an open mind to stay at the forefront of your career. I get huge satisfaction from helping people and making a difference in their lives; it's what I wake up for each day. The people who work for me tell me I'm just short of obsessed about being able to provide comfortable and calming experiences for my patients.

I put a lot of my energy into my practice—I love what I do. I'm 100% committed to learning and knowing all I can and translating that knowledge and experience into a better, healthier life for my patients.

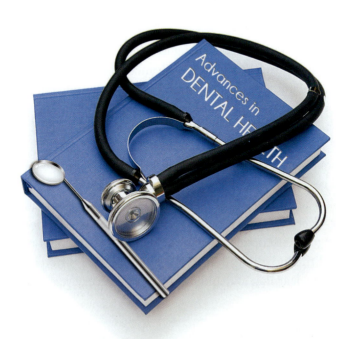

Chapter 4

I Became a Dentist because of a 12-Year-Old Boy in 1960s San Diego

I was playing dodgeball in the school yard when I fell. I got out of the way of the ball, but not the asphalt. I hit hard. There I was, face-down on the playground with a broken tooth, a bruised ego, and my mom rushing in to take me to the dentist. I'm not sure what my parents were thinking—either it was the least expensive or fastest solution or they were not offered choices—but I was given a silver front tooth.

It was ugly and clunky and it stood out like sore thumb—every budding teenager's nightmare. I was mortified. I became the guy who never smiled. I was hounded by kids taunting me, "There's Silver Tooth," "Hey Silver Tooth"—you get the idea. It wasn't fun. I never wanted to have my picture taken, either. The tooth negatively impacted my social life and how I felt about myself. It was a miserable time for me. I didn't want any other kid to have to go through that kind of humiliation—ever—and that motivated me to become a dentist, which led to a life of helping other people and seeking out leading-edge solutions to a variety of health challenges.

Fast forward almost 20 years to the early 1980s. My mother was diagnosed with metastatic lung cancer which resulted in her early death; she had just turned 50. As a medical professional, I was desperate to find answers and get information—to find a way to help my mom, if

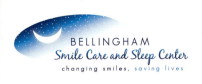

not to get better, at least to keep her from suffering so miserably. She was totally rung out, used up, exhausted, and sick—and I just didn't know what to do to help her. I felt pretty useless, standing by watching her endure treatment.

The experience with my mom lit a burning desire to find different ways to look at disease and the medical and dental professions. I've been open-minded my entire career continuously looking for better, easier, and more comfortable choices for my patients. I think when people are educated, they're empowered, so my goal is to offer information you might not find elsewhere.

My entire practice is driven by that one question I ask myself and my staff every single day we unlock our doors: What is best for our patients?

Perspective from Dr. Prager's Dental Hygienist:

"Dr. Prager is totally devoted to his practice and it shows up in so many positive ways for his patients and his staff. Our office works together as a team. He really invests the time and energy to make sure we're all informed, working together and that we know one another.

"He makes sure we do fun things outside the office so we bond and care about one another—because he feels that makes the office a great place to be and the patients feel that. He'll take us all to dinner, or on boat rides and other fun things that are great perks, but also really help us connect to one another so we bring that great camaraderie into the office. We have each other's backs and we pride ourselves in making sure the patients feel that same sense of fun and belonging. I've never had that in a work environment before. There's a real respect and we all want to pull our weight and do our part to make the practice thrive and the patients feel cared for and happy."

— Shawn M., Registered Dental Hygienist

Chapter 5

Does the Thought of Regular Checkups Stress You Out?

I know, you've heard it all your life—you need regular dental checkups. Yet, so many people put them off because they're afraid.

There have been some remarkable changes in dentistry in recent years. New technologies allow us to treat patients in ways that minimize fear and pain with procedures that are much less invasive and time consuming. I know if my patients are comfortable they are more likely to get treatment that keeps them healthy, and even prolong their life in some cases.

Have you ever felt apprehensive about going to the dentist? Anxious, even? Have you avoided the dentist altogether because you were afraid? Many people feel like Barbara Forss of Ferndale, WA did about visiting the dentist:

> "I never thought I'd actually look forward to coming to the dentist. I grew up in an era when dental visits were always associated with fear, noise, and pain. Dr. Prager has been my dentist for 12 years now and he is the most caring dentist I've ever met. His knowledge, equipment, techniques, and most of all his engaging demeanor are what make him the best of the best. I feel like I'm part of a nurturing, caring family.
>
> "My hygienist is totally awesome. I've been taught so much about the care and cleaning of my teeth and how it affects our overall health. Who knew a trip to the dentist could be fun?"

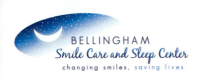

There is a better dental experience, where instead of being afraid you can actually be relaxed. I'm passionate about reducing—or better yet, eliminating—people's fear. I want to expand your view of what can be achieved by an up-to-date dental physician. Technology has changed our profession, making treatment easier and quicker for patients, with little or no pain.

"After years of avoiding dental offices because of past bad experiences, it finally reached the point where I had to face reality and take action before the damage to my teeth become irreversible.

"I'm so glad I chose Dr. Prager and his staff to guide me through the process. The atmosphere in his office is positive and encouraging and work that was done was virtually painless. The relief I feel at having dealt with this major issue and having it behind me is enormous. The anxiety that had ruled my thinking about dentists has been totally wiped out."

Ted Askew – Bellingham, WA

Chapter 6

Shock Factor—Oral Health Impacts Your Overall Health

Here's a shocking fact: Only 38% of Americans see a dentist regularly. That means a full 62% of the population—nearly two-thirds of Americans—aren't taking proper care of their oral health. You probably don't realize you put your overall health at risk when you don't have regular dental checkups. Ignoring problems in your mouth, whether mild or severe, can lead to greater problems and possibly, great expense.

And it's not just the health of your teeth that we look at. In my practice, I routinely help people with chronic headaches, migraines, sleep disorders, snoring, sleep apnea, and TMJ (jaw joint) problems—all problems related to teeth, muscles, ligaments, joints, and the anatomy of the head and neck.

> "People that keep their natural teeth live an average of 10 years longer than those that lose their teeth."
> – Dr. Charles Mayo, co-founder of the world famous Mayo Clinic

Here's something else that might surprise you: your oral health, literally the state of your mouth, offers clues about your overall health.

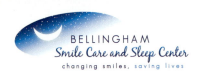

The mouth is the visible gateway to the rest of your body and reflects what is happening deep inside, things that might only otherwise be found with sophisticated (and expensive) testing or might be discovered when symptoms you can't ignore begin to appear.

It's not a stretch to say that your state of oral health can impact your life, your overall well-being, even how long you live!

Dentists like to talk about what we call the oral-systemic connection. Translated from "medical speak," it means there is a real connection between what happens in your mouth and diseases that you'll find throughout your entire system. Here are just a few of the risks you run by having poor oral health, according to the Mayo Clinic:

- Endocarditis. Endocarditis is an infection of the inner lining of your heart (endocardium). Endocarditis typically occurs when bacteria or other germs from another part of your body, such as your mouth, spread through your bloodstream and attach to damaged areas in your heart.

- Cardiovascular disease. Some research suggests that heart disease, clogged arteries, and stroke might be linked to the inflammation and infections that oral bacteria can cause.

- Pregnancy and birth. Periodontitis (gum and bone disease) has been linked to premature birth and low birth weight.

- Diabetes. Diabetes reduces the body's resistance to infection, putting the gums at risk. Gum disease appears to be more frequent and severe among people who have diabetes. Research shows that people who have gum disease have a harder time controlling their blood sugar levels.

- Alzheimer's disease. Tooth loss before age 35 and oral bacterial infection might be a risk factor for Alzheimer's disease.

- Pancreatic cancer as well as head and neck cancer have both been linked to oral bacteria.

Kind of an eye-opener, isn't it? Then, there's your teeth to consider and why keeping them healthy can make you happier, more attractive, and add years to your life. At The Bellingham Smile Care and Sleep Center we routinely improve lives, increase our patients' quality of life and their confidence.

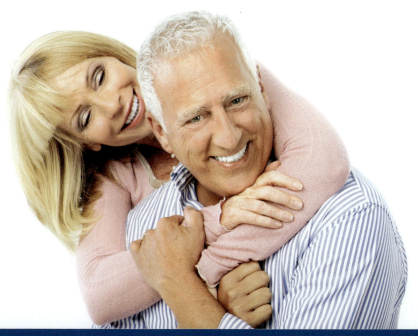

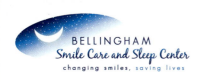

"She laughs at everything you say. Why? Because she has fine teeth." – Benjamin Franklin

From a very young age, Crystal Miner's teeth controlled her life. She never felt that anyone could truly understand just how psychologically painful her unattractive teeth were for her. On occasion she would forget how embarrassed she felt about her mouth until someone would ask her what happened to her or they'd look from her eyes to her mouth and she could see their shock register. It made her sick to her stomach.

Crystal likes to say that we gave her a second chance in life, that we made her look on the outside the beauty she always felt on the inside.

Crystal lived in fear of speaking to people or smiling—her teeth dramatically affected her personality and kept her from taking emotional risks. She actually even avoided going out sometimes, just to avoid interacting with people and feeling uncomfortable and embarrassed.

That's a lonely and painful way to live, something that's hard to understand if you haven't experienced it personally. Here's what Crystal said to us after just one visit and the cosmetic bonding that she says changed her life:

"Thank you from the bottom of my heart and from the smile on my face. My worries and anxiety have vanished. I feel content and no longer live with self-doubt. Dr Prager made me beautiful on my wedding day and I couldn't ask for more."

Crystal Miner – Bellingham, WA

Chapter 7

The Oral Health/Systemic Disease Connection

Numerous recent scientific studies indicate associations between oral health and a variety of general health conditions—including diabetes and heart disease. In response, the World Health Organization has integrated oral health into its chronic disease prevention efforts "as the risks to health are linked."

The American Dental Association recommends that dental visits begin no later than a child's first birthday to establish a "dental home." Dentists can provide guidance to children and parents, deliver preventive oral health services, and diagnose and treat dental disease in its earliest stages. This ongoing dental care will help both children and adults maintain optimal oral health throughout their lifetimes.

Dentists' areas of care include not only their patients' teeth and gums but also the muscles of the head, neck, and jaw, and the tongue, salivary glands, the nervous system of the head and neck, and other areas.

Dealing with common problems before they get out of control means you can spend less money on dental care, enjoy life more, and feel great knowing you're winning the battle on the frontline of your health care. Surely that's better than living with that nagging feeling that there's something you ought to be doing, but would rather avoid.

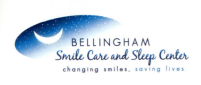

"I avoided going to the dentist for 6 years because of a very bad experience; I could not get numb enough. Apparently there are different kinds of Novocain—they are using one that works for me. The dental hygienist who did my deep tissue cleaning was wonderful.

"What could have been an awful, painful experience over several visits was not, because she is the best anyone could ever have. She has years of experience and is so warm and positive. I actually had fun seeing her. That is not the usual for a dental visit for me. I have no fear in their office. This is a miracle with my history! If there is a dental heaven, Dr. Prager's office and staff is it!"

Christina Kiemel – Mt. Vernon, WA

Chapter 8

"Dental Terror"—a Solution to Reduce or Even Eliminate Your Fear and Anxiety

I'm excited to tell you about a big game changer. We're the only practice in our corner of Northwestern Washington to offer it.

Introducing NuCalm - Imagine Enjoying Your Dental Appointment!

> "New ideas pass through three periods:
> 1. It can't be done.
> 2. It probably can be done, but it's not worth doing.
> 3. I knew it was a good idea all along."
>
> – Arthur C. Clarke

Really. Truly. I mean that sincerely. Enjoying your visit to the dentist can be a reality for you like it is for so many of our patients.

We all fear pain. In fact, fear of pain is one of the biggest human behavioral drivers. We're more motivated to avoid pain than anything else, including seeking pleasure. Your body is wired to avoid pain.

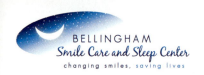

When you touch the burning stove, the pain warns you to back off or risk being burned. When you break a bone, the pain tells you to seek medical help that you need to heal.

Patients have come to associate pain with the dentist chair. They fear dental syringes—I don't use them. I'm a syringe-free dentist, but I still get patients profoundly numb because I use the high-tech dental Wand to numb their teeth (you'll learn a bit more about the Wand a bit later in the book). Patients will look at me with that edgy fear in their eyes and ask if I'm about to use the dreaded syringe, and I can say, "Nope, already numbed you; it'll kick in shortly."

Patients fear the pain of having their teeth drilled. I've seen more grown men and women cry—from fear and then from relief—when they learn that they can get routine dentistry done with total comfort and that we can actually relieve their anxiety and put them in a state of relaxation.

As promised, I'm going to share information that might surprise you—dental solutions for problems as diverse as migraine headaches, loose teeth you were told can't be saved, sleep apnea, snoring, and much more. I want you to read all that follows—a lot of good news—with an open mind, without part of your mind busy thinking, "Yeah, that

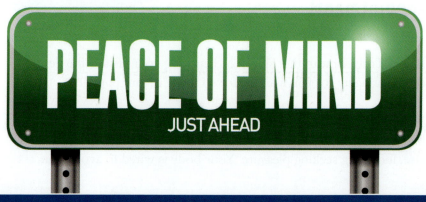

sounds good, but I'm terrified of going to the dentist." So, let's address your fear and anxiety first, put your mind at ease so you can stay open and so you will know—with absolute certainty—that together we can solve many of your health challenges while reducing your anxiety and calming your fear. Sound too good to be true? Read on . . .

Drug-Free and Powerful

NuCalm is a revolutionary drug-free approach to relaxation and anxiety reduction. You're probably familiar with laughing gas (nitrous oxide). It's commonly used in dentistry, but truth is, it can be dangerous, even toxic. Laughing gas has been associated with miscarriage and can be harmful for the dentist and dental assistants who breathe it all day long. Quite a few people say laughing gas nauseates them, and so naturally they don't want it.

Oral conscious sedation using prescription medications has some downsides, too. When you use conscious sedation, you have to eat a special diet and be driven to and from your appointment, so you need someone else who can take the time away from work or family to accompany you. Drugs can have negative side effects for some people, which are unpleasant at best. You lose an entire day recuperating while you wait for the drug to get out of your system. You can't work, drive, or concentrate, so you can't get right back to what you need to do. Even if the dental procedure is quick, the drugs take the same amount of time to wear off.

Enter NuCalm. Until fairly recently, NuCalm was used primarily to treat Post Traumatic Stress Disorder (PTSD) with veterans. It is also used in cardiology and oncology with heart and cancer patients, to calm them during treatment for conditions that we know cause stress. NuCalm is also being used by professional sports teams with their top-level athletes. In fact, there are some rumors that NuCalm is the "secret weapon" responsible for helping create the peak performance that has won some major league games. Keep your ears open about that one.

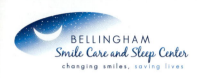

NuCalm and Dentistry—the Relaxing Approach

Today, a handful of elite dental practices are using NuCalm with phenomenal results. There is extensive training involved and it has to be the right type of practice. Our practice was honored to be chosen to be the very first in our corner of Northwestern Washington to offer NuCalm to create anxiety-free dental visits for our patients.

Thanks to research and our understanding of the connection between brain chemistry and the relaxation response, in four simple steps NuCalm induces a state of relaxation that can radically change your dental experience. Essentially, we recreate that delicious, safe, and peaceful sensation you experience right before you drift off to sleep at night. Time flies by, patients tell us they thought 15 or 20 minutes had elapsed after an hour in the chair—a fearless, anxiety-free, relaxing hour, I might add! Just imagine what a relief that would be.

NuCalm Step 1:

You chew two tablets that are natural supplements and amino acids. Both are natural neurotransmitters—messengers, if you will—produced by the brain when you're about to fall asleep at night; that delicious, relaxing feeling you have occurs because you produce these compounds. Their job is to "notify" your brain that

"The NuCalm is great! I don't think I would have been able to have my treatment without it." Robin White – Blaine, WA

relaxation is imminent, which causes you to begin to ease into the state of rejuvenating sleep.

NuCalm Step 2:
With patches behind your ear that produce a gentle Micro-current Stimulation (MCS), you achieve another layer of deep relaxation, and it's totally painless. MCS is an FDA-approved technique used for years to treat anxiety, post-traumatic stress syndrome, headaches, and migraines, and to produce relaxation. The light electro-current it delivers is similar to the current that "fires" all the cells in your body. Think of it as cancelling the flight-or-fight state that you feel when you're stressed or anxious. Instead of your body producing adrenaline so you get ratcheted up, the micro-current and amino acids create the lock and key connection that tells your brain to relax. This is about the time we see patients with a nice broad smile—they feel good, and so do we!

NuCalm Step 3:
The noise-cancelling headphones you're fitted with are playing relaxing music layered with neuro-acoustic software. This synchronizes your brain into an alpha state, the first stage of sleep. You can still hear and respond, but you are relaxed and peaceful. You are never asleep, but you are in a state of reduced anxiety and extreme relaxation.

NuCalm Step 4:
We give you dark glasses to block out any visual stimuli, allowing you to stay completely and totally relaxed.

I've seen a lot of new technology over the years and we have some techniques we can use to save our patients' natural teeth and treat

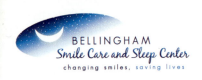

a whole range of health problems. But—and this is a big BUT—if patients are too terrified to come in and see us, we can't help them. And, if we can't help them, their problems get worse. I feel terrible when I see patients who come in because they're at a point where they just can't avoid their problem any longer. That usually means they've been troubled or have been suffering for a while. Why do they wait? Because most of them had bad experiences and they're terrified. I'll never forget the first time I used NuCalm on a patient for a dental

Jeff Goodman came in to see us for the first time a few years back. He was no stranger to crowns, having had three done previously. He told us that being injected with a hypodermic needle was excruciating for him and his previous experiences left him feeling like he'd been run over by a truck. He put it this way: "The next day you couldn't touch me with a powder puff I was so sore." At his previous dental office, he was given temporaries during that treatment and was told they wouldn't feel right, but he'd only have to wear them for three weeks. Jeff said, "It was like chewing on a batch of gravel for three weeks—my tongue looked like hamburger."

You can imagine that Jeff was not running into our office super excited about dental work. Jeff did in fact need crowns, but here's what he told us after having crowns done in our office:

"I'd have to say I'd do all those others again under your care if it would erase the memory of how traumatic those first three times at the other dental office were. The numbing procedure is one of the worst, if not THE worst part for me, but your procedure was almost without any sensation. Instead of feeling run over by a truck, I was feeling normal the same evening and didn't need to take any Tylenol. The next day I was just a little sore but had no need for pain relief. Needless to say, I'm a fan and truly grateful to have a dentist I won't dread going to!"

procedure. Sue was terrified of dental work; she literally cried when she came into the office. She was so nervous she wouldn't even let me examine her teeth; she was freaked out. The only reason she showed up was because she needed a procedure she couldn't put off. She was keen to try NuCalm when we told her about it.

She was totally and completely relaxed and calm and when the exam and procedure was over and we removed the glasses and headphones, she looked surprised and asked me "Are you done already? Wow. I feel great, like I had a power nap. You already did the work?" She was blown away and so was I. I knew it would be a huge breakthrough for other patients too.

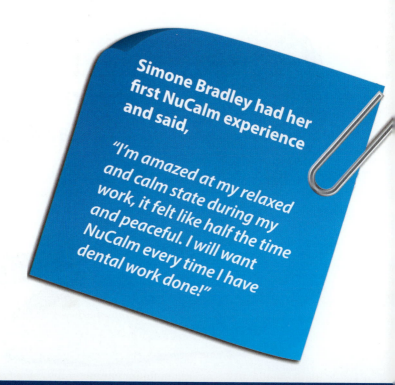

Simone Bradley had her first NuCalm experience and said,

"I'm amazed at my relaxed and calm state during my work, it felt like half the time and peaceful. I will want NuCalm every time I have dental work done!"

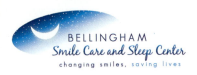

> "I'm surprised how relaxed I felt during the appointment using NuCalm. It was a very good experience! I will be recommending NuCalm to my family and friends."
> Maria Matei – Ferndale, WA

NuCalm can be used with every procedure. Simple, easy, effective. Imagine leaving the dental chair feeling refreshed and relaxed instead of wrung out and relieved that it's over and you're done!

I'd like you to keep NuCalm in mind as you read—telling yourself that now EVERY dental procedure can be done anxiety-free and in a state of total relaxation.

Dr. Prager in "Nu-Calm Land"

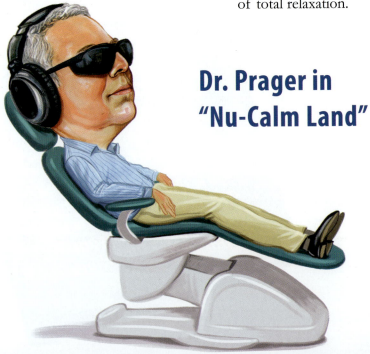

Chapter 9

Gum Disease and Tooth Loss—an Innovative, Smart, and Comfortable Solution

"In all things it is better to hope than to despair."
– Johan Wolfgang Von Goethe

Gum and bone (periodontal) disease, which is the most common adult dental problem and the major cause of tooth loss—more so than cavities, by the way—is typically treated by painful invasive surgery that takes a long time to recover from. That's why so many people with moderate to severe disease put off treatment.

In fact many people avoid dealing with gum disease until they are in so much pain and/or their teeth are so loose that they are forced to seek help.
I've seen so many patients over the years who came to me just devastated because they had gum and bone disease. Their dentist didn't give them any hope, usually telling them they were going to lose teeth—several teeth, sometimes all their teeth—and that's hard news to hear.

It's awful being told, "You've got gum disease . . . you'll need surgery . . . you're going to lose your teeth . . . they'll give you the number

> "Several years ago I had minor gum surgery which resulted in serious gum shrinkage. I began having my teeth cleaned every three to four months. The technique involved sharp prongs and flushing water. I was swallowing huge amounts of what I assume was bacteria-laden water and I always had very sore, tender gums from the probes. Frequently, my gums would just quiet down when it was time for another cleaning. I pestered my dentist with requests for alternative and different solutions but he had none.
>
> "Six months after my dental coverage was terminated because of retirement, my dentist advised me he did not know what to do with my teeth anymore because they were in such awful condition. I was told extraction and full dentures were inevitable for me.
>
> "It was like a miracle that I heard Dr. Prager's ad on the radio. I made an appointment and proceeded with treatment. I was astonished at how easy it was for me. There was no pain! During the longer appointments I even caught myself almost falling asleep! Dr. Prager and his staff are amazing. They are friendly, quite efficient, and fast. My follow-up appointments are showing great results and healing and I am so grateful for the opportunity to get such excellent care with the best technology and expertise available. Dr. Prager saved my teeth! My only regret is that I didn't find Dr. Prager and his office earlier."
>
> **Fran Schultze - Surrey, British Columbia, Canada**

of the gum surgeon (periodontist) at the front desk." Patients can feel confused, even devastated. They don't feel like they have options and it can be a frightening time. The last thing you want is to feel like you're a case to solve, not a person with feelings, fears, and phobias. Compassion goes a long way to helping put patients at ease. Giving them options is critically important.

Some dentists see gum disease or gum pockets and they want to rip teeth out and put in implants. Sometimes I think my colleagues got together and decided we're all experiencing a titanium deficiency, so they want to put in artificial titanium tooth roots and cure the shortage for everyone.

Surgery and implants are expensive, potentially painful, and they don't save teeth. I believe my job as a dentist is to give people hope and treat them with compassion. I think it's important to explore every option to save teeth and avoid surgery when possible. I believe your best implant is your own natural tooth and I take great pride in being able to save teeth that other dentists thought should be extracted.

Let's choose the least invasive and best value treatment that will solve the problem. If it means going to the time and expense of learning new techniques and purchasing the equipment to perform them so I can save my patient's teeth, let's do that.

Let's do whatever it takes to give our patients HOPE and save their natural teeth.

As I mentioned earlier, gum (periodontal) disease is the most common reason adults lose teeth—much more common than losing them from cavities. In our office we use our Periolase Laser to perform LANAP® (Laser Assisted New Attachment Procedure) to treat gum disease—a sophisticated laser technology that works brilliantly well, saves teeth and keeps so many patients from undergoing painful surgery and helps them avoid dentures and/or implants. LANAP® took Suzanne Leech from devastation to hope:

> "A few weeks before my 50th birthday I was hiking and had a bad fall. I displaced and chipped two of my front teeth and needed to see a dentist. After the exam the dentist came in and I was expecting to hear how she was going to repair my teeth. Instead, I was told I had advanced periodontal disease and would need to have ALL my teeth extracted and be fitted for dentures. After the shock wore off I asked about alternatives and was told flat out there weren't any..."

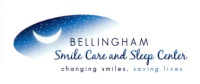

"The dentist went on to tell me that I had no time to lose, I had passed a tipping point and really had to do this immediately before it impacted my overall long term health—the longer I waited, the greater the risk.

"I was totally devastated. I went to a really dark place. I was literally having nightmares about being toothless. I would wake up panicked in the middle of the night. I had neglected dentistry for 20 years; I had a lifelong fear of dentistry. I was angry at myself because ultimately this was preventable, so the blame rested squarely on my shoulders.

"I made an appointment with an extraction specialist and I kept thinking about all the wonderful advances we hear about almost every day in medicine. Surely there had to be some dental advance that would help me. I got online and read about LANAP®. At that time is was experimental but people were reporting good results from treatment. Then I happened to come across a flyer about Dr. Prager and I went to his website to check him out and learned he was the only dentist performing LANAP® in the entire Pacific Northwestern corner of Washington and he was right here in Bellingham!

"I went in hopeless and was immediately given hope. Dr. Prager was honest with me, saying that he wasn't sure he could save all my teeth, but he was confident he could save most of them. I'll never forget what he said to me: "We're embarking on a great adventure together." I left the office feeling elated and filled with hope.

"I experienced no pain or discomfort that I always associated with dentistry. The LANAP® was completed in two visits and six months later Dr. Prager told me I would be able to keep all my teeth. I didn't experience any of the pain or discomfort I associated with dentistry for decades.

"Dr. Prager took all the time I needed; he's a perfectionist. And it's a great experience every time you walk through the door. Everyone knows your name, they're friendly, and you don't wait around—they're waiting for you when you arrive!

"I've become an advocate for dental care—I don't want anyone else to put off seeing a dentist and getting the care they need, especially now that I know it can be an easy experience where you're well taken care of and it's not the misery and fear I once knew." **Suzanne Leech – Bellingham, WA**

Saving Suzanne's natural teeth made the world of difference for her. She really did go from devastation to being happy, and in a way, getting her life back. I've had patients come to me from as far away as Kotzebue, Alaska (above the Arctic Circle) and Los Angeles, CA (and everywhere in between) to be treated with LANAP®. It's that remarkable a treatment; people actually seek it out once they know it's a viable alternative to gum surgery and that it can save their natural teeth and help them avoid dentures, partials, or dental implants.

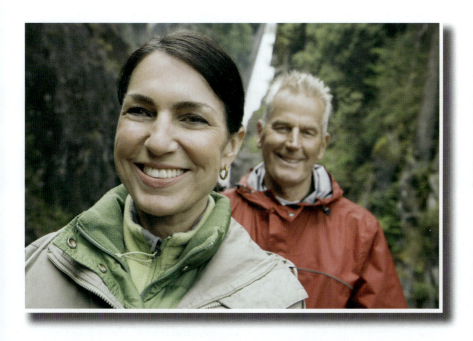

Here's a professional perspective on LANAP® vs. gum surgery:

"I'm a dental hygienist and I've spent most of my career working for a periodontist, assisting in gum surgeries, among other things. In performing surgery for gum disease we had to remove so much gum tissue and that often caused more root exposure. The root is extremely sensitive, so exposure can be really uncomfortable. Typically there's a lot of healing time involved with traditional gum surgery—and that's not pleasant for most patients. Patients often experienced bone loss and we had to replace their bone with synthetic or animal bone—it's fairly involved, as you can imagine.

"I had never heard of LANAP® treatment, so when I came to work for Dr. Prager I was amazed to see what could be accomplished with the Periolase laser. I was taught in hygienist school that when you lose bone you can't ever get it back, but the laser actually stimulates and promotes bone growth—I was amazed by that. I've seen the x-rays of patients before and after LANAP® and there is definitely more bone there. Not only does the laser rid the patient of disease, it actually helps them be healthier! And gum surgery recovery can be long and painful; with laser, it just isn't.

"I got to wondering why more people don't use this treatment. I think that for many dentists, taking on something new like LANAP® is probably a bit scary; it's something new and different and it takes a big investment of time and money to learn the process and invest in the equipment. People get set in their ways. Dr. Prager took the time to invest in his practice and LANAP® specifically, and that has made a huge difference for his patients."

Shawn M., Registered Dental Hygienist

Chapter 10

Gum Disease Treatment without Invasive Surgery— LANAP® Is Good News

Sadly, most general dentists prefer to refer patients to a periodontist—meaning, they view gum amputation surgery as the first (and perhaps only) solution for moderate to severe gum disease . My first line of defense is not only a much simpler and easier solution, but one of greater value and greater comfort.

Let's face it, it's the rare general dentist that wants to send you to another general dentist and risk losing you as a patient. I respect that and I understand it completely. Yet, I have to ask:

What's best for the patient? That should be the deciding factor.

> "All truth passes through three stages: First it is ridiculed. Second it is violently opposed. Third it is accepted as being self-evident."
> – Arthur Schopenhauer

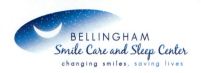

How LANAP® Works to Treat Gum Disease and Why It's a Great Option

A tiny laser fiber (about the thickness of three hairs) is inserted between the tooth and the gum, and the laser effectively clears the infection away. Think of LANAP® like erasing a blackboard—there's no cutting, no stitches, and none of the pain that goes along with surgery. You're comfortable during the procedure and comfortable when it's over.

LANAP® is less time consuming than surgery with less follow-up needed. You save time, money, aggravation, gum tissue, and you're more comfortable—kind of a no-brainer, don't you think? And, because the recovery period is less than 24 hours, you won't miss time from work or other activities.

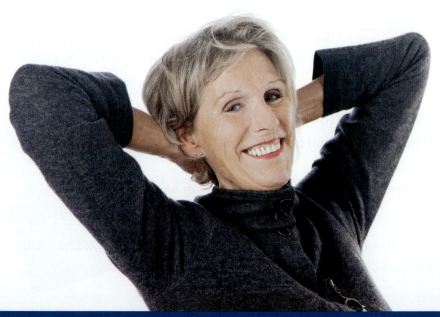

When Pandora came to see us she was very shy and even seemed a bit withdrawn. She hardly talked and when she did, she held her hand in front of her mouth. Her gums were terribly infected; she was suffering from severe gum and bone disease. We treated her gum disease with LANAP® and she literally cried with gratitude when we saved her teeth and rid her of infection. She had previously been told there was no hope for her teeth and dentures were her only choice.

After we finished and everything had healed, she told me and my staff that she was in retail and she could hardly talk to people and never smiled—she hated how her teeth looked. I told her that now that we had saved her own natural teeth, we could change the look of her teeth, that dental porcelain veneers would give her a brand new smile.

She was thrilled by the idea. In our office we make custom acrylic temporaries from a wax mock-up model. We have patients wear them home to show to family and friends and to look at them in the mirror over a few days to see what they think.

Pandora's husband was actually moved to tears when she came home with her temporaries. He was blown away by how different she looked, but also by how happy and relieved she was to have a brand new smile—even with just the acrylic temporaries.

After getting her permanent veneers, Pandora's personality changed completely. She went from introvert to very talkative. She was comfortable interacting with people and her confidence was through the roof. Pandora was like a different person; no one in our office could believe it. We love making a difference in our patients' lives.

All that from a saved mouth. And the irony? Other dentists had told her there was no hope and had recommended pulling all her teeth and giving her dentures or full-mouth titanium root implants.

Gum disease is the most common adult dental condition. Our Periolase laser saves teeth that would otherwise be lost. This is modern dentistry at its best and as you can see, it can be life changing.

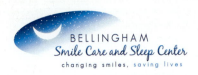
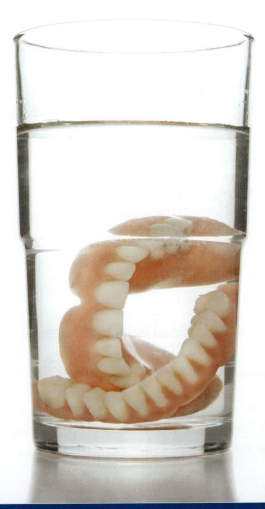

Chapter 11

Your Own Teeth Are Your Best Teeth—You Want to Keep Them!

Over my entire career and by learning about the leading-edge technology of the time—and boy, has it changed a lot in the last two decades—I've searched for ways to help my patients keep their God-given teeth, which when possible is ALWAYS the best option.

As I said before, I think too many dentists today are "crazy for implants." Sometimes, implants are the only solution. But they should never be the default solution. It's a sad fact that today most dentists don't make a big effort to try and save natural teeth. In our office, we only treat patients with implants when saving natural teeth isn't an option.

I have techniques and technology for saving your teeth that many of my colleagues aren't trained in—some don't even know they exist!

Believe Me, You Want to Keep Your Own Natural Teeth

I cannot say this strongly enough or often enough: your own natural teeth are the best teeth and keeping them should be the first priority of dental care and treatment.

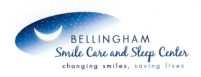

Truth is, more teeth are being extracted today than ever before. That's a dirty little secret no one wants you to know. Most dentists don't try and save teeth. And they don't warn you that when you lose teeth, it can permanently change your face. You lose face bone and jaw bone when you lose teeth; wow did anyone ever tell you that? Your face caves in where the missing teeth were, so your face changes shape. What could be worse than looking in the mirror after a dental procedure that was supposed to help you and the person looking back not only looks instantly older, but doesn't look like you?

Your mouth is so important. Think about this for a moment. You could live without a limb—not that you would want to—but many people do and prosthetics and technology are making steady advancements to make sustaining injuries and loss of limbs more manageable than ever before.

You can't, however, live without a functioning mouth with the ability to swallow, breathe, or chew. Stop breathing and it's game over. And you can't sustain life without eating or drinking water.

All of these functions require using your mouth. And, your brain is structured such that 40% of all the input to your brain comes from your lower face and jaw muscle complex. This area is remarkable when you consider that your entire body is made up of muscles and nerves. That's tremendous influence coming through the specific part of the brain that deals with the upper and lower jaws and the muscles that move the jaw. Your mouth, teeth, tongue, and the bones and muscles in your face play a hugely important role in your overall health. It's that important.

Five Tightly Guarded, Closely Held Secrets

. . . that most dentists don't want you to know. But if you follow all Five Secrets, they will allow you to save your natural teeth for your lifetime.

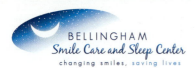
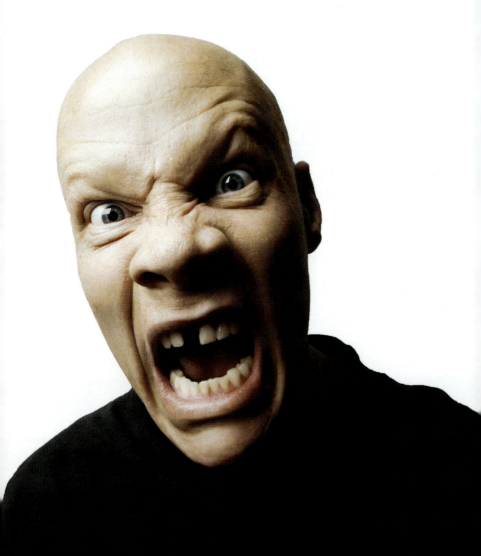

Secret #1

Why Each Tooth Is Critically Important—If You Lose a Tooth, Replace it!

Have you ever seen someone with missing teeth? You might notice how they put their hand to their mouth when they laugh or smile, or they don't smile much because they're embarrassed. Our smile conveys a lot about who we are. It's said that 90% of human communication is received and interpreted through body language and it begins with the smile. It's the way that we connect to others and establish rapport.

How your smile looks and feels matters. And, when you feel good about your smile, you become empowered, no longer a victim. That's what we can do for people—empower them to feel better about themselves and more confident.

Losing a tooth and not replacing it leads to losing a second and then a third tooth, further compromising your looks, the structural integrity of your mouth, and your health. You force the remaining teeth to work much harder than they were designed to.

Teeth are built to work as a team. When you have a missing tooth, your other teeth are more likely to break down, move, or change position. Think of it as a cascading, or domino effect. If you lose all your back teeth—guess what? You can't chew with just your upper and lower six front teeth. It's game over (teeth-wise) if that happens.

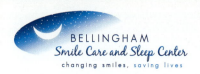

The solution is to replace ANY missing tooth immediately, especially back teeth (except wisdom teeth). Otherwise, you'll experience the dreaded domino effect, losing additional teeth and destabilizing your bite. That can lead to potentially painful jaw joint problems, bite problems, headaches, sleep problems, and a future of dental problems and expense.

The secret is to replace missing teeth—as soon as possible so you can save your other teeth and stay healthy.

Secret #2

You Don't Know the 60/40 Rule

When you wash your hair, do you only wash 60% and leave the rest dry and dirty? Do you wax only 60% of your car or cut 60% of your lawn? How about serving only 60% of dinner? Or doing 60% of your job at work? That'll get you fired!

You brush your teeth, right? Get this—no matter what type of toothbrush you use and what kind of toothpaste, you're only cleaning 60% of your teeth surfaces. Every time you brush, it's a job only 60% completed. Even the most conscientious brushers can't do 100% of the job. You'd be missing what's BETWEEN your teeth . . . kind of like cleaning the top and bottom of the fork you used for dinner, but leaving the food stuck between the tines—ick!

What's worse is that most of the problems dentists see are in that 40% that you're missing. There are a number of things you can do to take better care of your teeth. Flossing daily is certainly one of them (I know, no one's favorite task).

We offer our patients a solution that they like much better. And, if you like it better, guess what? You do it! Our patients are introduced to a tool called the Hydro Floss. It's water under pressure, it feels great and it gets deeper than flossing ever could and most important—it's easy to use and very affordable. We order special cleaning tips for our patients for extra comfort and effectiveness. With Hydro Floss you can great results without using the floss so many people dread.

No flossing lectures in our office—ever.

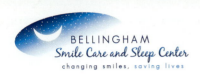
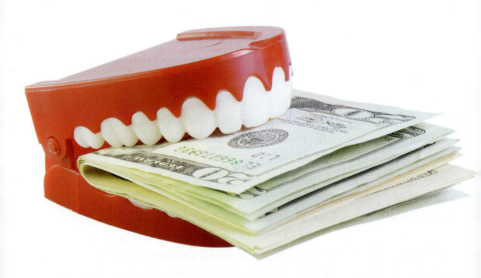

Secret #3

Dentistry Isn't Expensive but Dental Neglect Is

Because so many people are terrified of seeing the dentist, they don't show up until they're in pain, have a serious problem, have an emergency (like an accident), or they can't stand the way their smile looks and they want a beautiful healthy smile and to look more attractive.

I see people who have mouths ravaged by cavities and/or gum and bone infection, some are in pain, others just concerned. They've neglected their oral health and now that they're ready to do something about it they are absolutely shocked by the cost of getting their mouth into a healthy state.

The big secret here: dental care isn't expensive, but dental neglect can end up being quite costly.

What could have been treated with a simple and small tooth-colored filling, now requires root canal treatment and a reinforced post and crown—costly and time consuming procedures—but at that point, there's just no other solution.

What could have been taken care of with routine and regular professional cleaning now requires multiple visits because we're treating advanced bone and gum disease. There is good news in this frightening equation though—we have helped hundreds upon hundreds of people

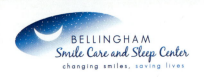

rebuild their mouths to excellent health and now they only need very minimal and cost-effective maintenance to stay healthy. Modern dentistry has a phenomenal preventive component.

In our office, we do everything we can to offer comfortable payment options and plans to our patients. Some are long term and others are interest-free. We aim to make our services affordable and our care accessible.

A WORD HERE ABOUT THE COST OF STAYING HEALTHY.

I believe it's important not to make decisions based on cost, but rather on value. The cheapest solution isn't always the best solution and you only have one set of teeth (see the "dental vacation" section that follows!). You can never replace your natural God-given teeth and since you've read this far, I hope you understand just how critically important that is.

Our goal at The Bellingham Smile Care and Sleep Center is to give superior value and top-notch quality and service. We work hard to find solutions that work for you. That includes offering a range of solutions to challenges you might not even think (first) of a dentist to solve.

Secret #4

Only Two Things Cause Tooth Loss—Control 'Em and You'll Keep 'Em

There are only two menaces standing between keeping your teeth in your mouth or looking at them in your hand: bacteria and stress. We all have bacteria in our mouths—that's how we're designed. However, the bad bacteria can get out of balance and wreak havoc with your health. Cavities and gum and bone disease are both caused by bacteria and the toxins they produce.

Bacterial balance can get out of whack a number of ways: if you have a less-than-healthy diet, take drugs, get run down, and by not removing bacteria through regular dental visits and careful care at home. The result isn't pretty. Your teeth can dissolve away from cavities and your jaw bone can dissolve from periodontal disease. Ouch.

Stress in your mouth may be a bit different than the stress you're used to thinking about. The main type of oral stress comes from the (literally) hundreds of pounds of pressure your jaw exerts when you chew or grind or clench. When these forces get out of balance, you'll break teeth or wear them down to "nubbins."

There's another stress you want to be aware of—acid stress. Acid stress is often caused by drinking fizzy drinks and beverages—even from too much fruit juice. Too much acid in your food or drink can draw calcium out of your teeth, causing them to erode—literally wash away.

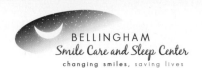

Stress from excessive grinding, gritting, clenching or gnashing of your teeth can cause jaw joint and muscle aches and can also cause your teeth to loosen or wear down to the bone. You don't want either of these to happen.

What can you do? Replace broken teeth right away so you keep your "team" of teeth intact and don't create any extra harming force on the remaining teeth. Keep your teeth clean through regular maintenance at home and regular dental visits to keep bacteria healthy and get rid of the bad bacteria. Switch your diet from acid-based to a more alkaline diet. Remember the old saying, an ounce of prevention is better than a pound of cure? There you have it.

Secret #5

Dental Insurance Is NOT What You Think It Is

Dental insurance is kind of an odd term—an oxymoron really. Why? Because it's not really insurance. It's actually a partial reimbursement program with very strict preset limits and exclusions. Unlike traditional insurance like auto or medical insurance that covers you in case of a loss, all dental insurance does is pay a portion of dental expenses up to a preset limit.

Dental insurance came into being about 40 years ago and sadly, nothing much has changed since then, including how much is paid—$1000 yearly maximum then and $1000 yearly maximum now! Forty years ago the average car cost $3,650 and a gallon of gas was 40 cents. Today the average car costs over $17,000. You get the idea.

If your mouth is unhealthy, $1000 won't go very far. However, it's only fair to say that it does help to maintain an already healthy mouth.

Here's the problem. People suffer in agony with tooth problems and they say, "I can't or won't go to the dentist because I don't have dental insurance." So they wait until they have insurance and then are devastated to learn $1000 doesn't cover the work they need—which is more expensive because they've put off treatment for so long. Or, they wait until their situation becomes so serious that they have no choice. Now they're in pain and probably spending more than they would have if they'd dealt with the problem sooner, or better yet, didn't neglect

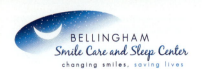

their teeth because they didn't have the "mythical dental insurance." Bad news? Dental insurance is not adequate for solving complex problems and years of neglect—it's just not designed for that.

Good news? In our office, we do everything we can to offer comfortable payment options and plans to our patients. Some are long term and some are interest-free. We aim to make our services affordable and our care accessible.

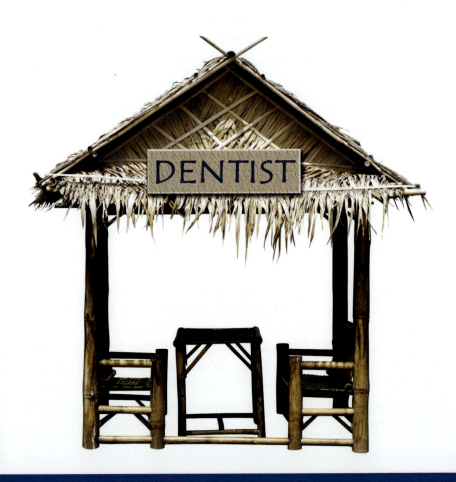

BONUS Secret

The Real Truth About "Dental Vacations"

Have you heard about dental vacations? Dental and medical vacations are popular at the moment.

You get a package—inexpensive medical care in a foreign country followed by some exotic travel. People get excited because it's cheap and it seems like a great way to kill the proverbial two birds with one stone: get something you need to do taken care of cheap and do something fun you want to do—travel—in the bargain.

Wait! Don't sign up without hearing this: it can cost you more—way more—in the long run. I've had people come in who want me to fix the dental work done on their "dental vacations." This is dentistry they've have had done all over the world—Mexico, China, Poland, Russia, Costa Rica, Colombia, Japan, England, and many other countries.

I've seen crowns and bridges fit so poorly that teeth and gums were completely ruined. Imagine patients sitting in my chair crying because their beautiful teeth are destroyed and now they're going to have to spend money to save them—the money they were trying to avoid spending in the first place—all after taking a "dental vacation." And they can't go back. A lot of people's teeth (and health) were damaged so badly there's no way they can be restored—that's a huge price to pay. What seemed like a great and economical idea turns out to be a costly nightmare—in terms of health and finances. Avoid this option—at any and all costs.

There you have it.
Five (and a bonus) simple secrets that if you follow, will without a doubt, allow you to keep your natural teeth for a lifetime.

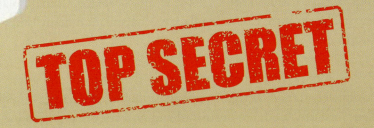

Chapter 12

Does Snoring Drive You or Your Bed Partner Crazy?

"Laugh and the world laughs with you. Snore and you sleep alone." – Anthony Burgess

Snoring might just seem like a mildly annoying interruption or a reason you occasionally or even regularly lose sleep—especially if you're the person who sleeps with the snorer. Hear this: not many people realize snoring can be very dangerous, even life-threatening in some cases. Most people who snore also suffer from some form of obstructive sleep apnea, but they don't know it. Snoring can be an indicator that you might stop breathing many times an hour during the night! Snoring on a frequent or regular basis has also been directly associated with stroke.

Dangerous symptoms of snoring to be aware of:

- Waking up with a very sore or dry throat
- Sleepiness or lack of energy during the day
- Teeth grinding . . . teeth clenching
- Occasionally waking up with a choking or gasping sensation
- Sleepiness while driving or watching television
- Morning headaches, restless sleep, constant yawning
- Forgetfulness, mood changes, and a decreased interest in sex
- Feeling like you could use an hour or two more sleep when you wake in the morning
- Recurrent awakenings or insomnia

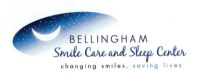

Snoring might not just be annoying and keeping you from getting a good night's sleep. And sleep may just be more important than you realize. We're designed to sleep and let our bodies and minds regenerate.

Sleep reduces stress, helps regulate weight, sharpens attention (note to parents: a good night's sleep could result in better grades), spurs creativity, and improves memory. Getting a good night's rest is critically important to your health and your quality of life.

RESEARCHERS AT THE UNIVERSITY OF CHICAGO found that dieters who were well rested lost more fat—56% more weight lost—than those who were sleep deprived, who lost more muscle mass. (They shed similar amounts of total weight regardless of sleep.) Dieters in the study also felt hungrier when they got less sleep. Sleep and metabolism are controlled by the same sectors of the brain. When you are sleepy, certain hormones go up in your blood and those same hormones drive appetite.

Chapter 13

Snoring Is a Literal Wake-Up Call —the Message? Something Is Wrong!

Snoring creates a vibration in the throat that causes plaque to accumulate in the carotid arteries—the large arteries in your neck that supply blood to the brain. The more junk you have in those arteries, the higher your risk for stroke. And, did you know that snoring is the number one medical cause for divorce? Untreated snoring can lead to sleep apnea—so treating snoring can save your life and your marriage.

It's important to understand that snoring can be an early sign of sleep apnea—a condition that's very important to treat.

And, you don't want to treat snoring without knowing if you or your bed partner has sleep apnea. Why? If you treat the snoring without getting a proper test from a certified sleep physician you could still have sleep apnea (where you stop breathing many times during the night) that's left untreated. This is not something to mess around with! You'll understand exactly why when you read the next section on sleep apnea.

Beware: There are dentists who will make "snore appliances" that may help reduce or eliminate snoring, without first determining whether you do, indeed, have sleep apnea. Before you get a snore

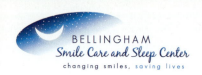

appliance, you really want to have a sleep study done and make sure it's read by a certified sleep physician—to diagnose if you have sleep apnea.

If you stop snoring while using a snore appliance made by an unenlightened dentist (or order one off the Internet) and aren't tested, there's a strong possibility that you are not receiving enough oxygen during the night, due to underlying sleep apnea. Let me say it loud and clear—that could put you on a course for an early death.

A prime example is the former manager for the Seattle Mariners who had a stroke, and it turned out it was related to undiagnosed sleep apnea. Please don't let snoring and stopping breathing go undiagnosed!

Chapter 14

Sleep Apnea Is a Serious Sleep Disorder with Many Potential Health Hazards

Eighty million Americans suffer from some form of Sleep Disordered Breathing—of which obstructive sleep apnea is the most common. Have you or someone you love been diagnosed with sleep apnea? Perhaps you think you might have sleep apnea but aren't sure. Snoring and sleep apnea are on the same continuum, and as you read in the previous section, snoring can be a precursor and is often an indicator that sleep apnea exists.

To determine if you have obstructive sleep apnea, you need to have a sleep test. Sleep tests can be administered in a medical facility, or you can have a sleep test at home—either way, the test must be analyzed by a certified sleep physician. Once you've had a sleep test (and we can give you information on how, when, and where to have that done) we'll know exactly what we're dealing with.

What Exactly Is Sleep Apnea?

Obstructive Sleep Apnea occurs when a patient's normal sleep is interrupted due to inadequate oxygen levels in the blood. When you don't have enough oxygen getting to your brain, your body triggers

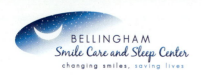

your fight or flight response. Imagine your body responding as if you've seen a tiger in the wild. If the tiger is going to chase you, you need the glucose in your muscles to help you run. Your fight or flight response kicks in and produces adrenaline from your adrenals and puts the glucose into your blood. Your heart races and your blood pressure increases. You're ready to avoid the predator to survive.

You don't need to run—you're sleeping! The first job of your brain stem is to keep you alive, so it constantly monitors to see if you have enough oxygen (it actually measures CO_2 levels which fluctuate inversely to oxygen levels). If you don't, you go into "fight or flight" and over the course of the night you become exhausted, repeating this process over and over again. This response can occur up to 100 times an hour in severe cases of sleep apnea. A mild case of sleep apnea might cause you to repeat this process up to 15 times in an hour, and in a moderate case, 15–30 times in an hour. And, untreated apnea always gets worse.

People with sleep apnea awaken (go from deep sleep to light sleep) frequently during the night, gasping for breath in order to restart their breathing process and restore their depleted oxygen.

These breathing pauses and reduced blood oxygen levels can strain the heart and cardiovascular system and increase the risk of cardiovascular disease. Stopping breathing or struggling to breathe strangulates your organs, including your heart and brain as well as other vital organs. Because your sleep is fragmented, you don't rest or feel rejuvenated. You wake exhausted instead of revitalized. It's disruptive at best and totally debilitating at worst.

Sleep apnea can be upsetting for the sufferers and for their bed partners whose sleep is also being constantly interrupted. Sleep apnea symptoms can include feeling tired upon waking, headaches, and a frustrating battle with fatigue throughout the day. Many sufferers grind their teeth, snore loudly, and feel irritable—not pleasant for anyone. They are slowly being robbed of their vitality night after night, week after week, and year after year, and the great majority of them don't know it.

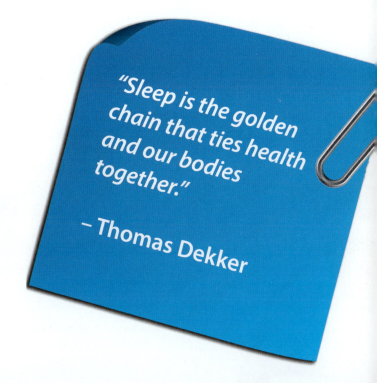

"Sleep is the golden chain that ties health and our bodies together."

– Thomas Dekker

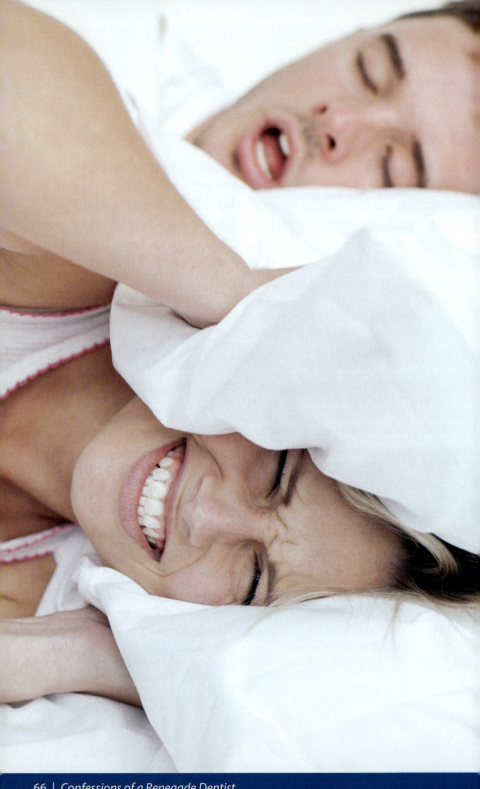

Chapter 15

How Do You Know If You Have Sleep Apnea?

You can't tell if you're suffering from sleep apnea because you're only semi-conscious at the time you'd be aware of the symptoms. Your sleep partner may be aware of your symptoms and they may be suffering from a lack of sleep while your symptoms wake them throughout the night. In fact, sleep apnea forces many partners into separate rooms—not a happy situation for many people.

Symptoms of Sleep Apnea to Look For:

- Sleepiness or lack of energy during the day
- Loud snoring and/or waking up with a very sore or dry throat
- Teeth grinding or teeth gnashing
- Occasionally waking up with a choking or gasping sensation
- Feeling sleepy while driving or watching television
- Morning headaches, restless sleep, constant yawning
- Forgetfulness and mood changes
- Decreased interest in sex, erectile dysfunction
- Not feeling rested when you wake in the morning
- Frequent waking during the night or insomnia

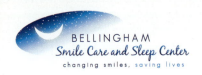

Sleep apnea is not something to ignore either. Untreated sleep apnea can increase your risk of high blood pressure, heart attack, stroke and early death. The average age of death of an untreated sleep apneic is 55 years of age! Sleep apnea and chronic low levels of oxygen in your blood can also contribute to:

- Muscle pain
- "Restless Leg Syndrome"
- Increased risk of depression
- Weight gain
- Diabetes
- Memory and concentration impairment
- Mood swings and/or temperamental behavior
- Fibromyalgia, pain in joints, muscles and tendons
- Hypertension (high blood pressure)
- Impotence
- Loss of short-term memory
- Gastric reflux
- Stroke
- Intellectual deterioration
- Insomnia
- Congestive heart failure
- Coronary artery disease

> "A good laugh and a long sleep are the best cures in the doctor's book." – Irish Proverb

Chapter 16

There Are Only Four Treatments for Sleep Apnea

There are no drugs or medicines that treat sleep apnea. Obstructive sleep apnea is a mechanical blockage of the throat causing oxygen levels to plummet, threatening your life and . . .

The Only Four Treatments Are:

1. CPAP (continuous positive airway pressure mask). This is the most commonly prescribed treatment for obstructive sleep apnea and it's very effective if it is used. Trouble is, studies continue to reveal that up to 50% of CPAP machines are abandoned, discarded or aren't used very much. If your CPAP is sitting at the bottom of your closet, it's not doing you or your sleep apnea any good.

2. Specialized oral appliances—more about this in a moment.

3. Throat Surgery—where part of your throat (soft palate) and associated structures are cut out—this is very painful and doesn't have a very high success rate. And if the surgery doesn't work, you can't get those parts of your throat back.

4. Tracheostomy—a hole is made under you voice box and plastic tube is inserted for you to breathe through. Don't laugh. This is the only 100% successful treatment for obstructive sleep apnea—but I've never been able to get anyone to go for it!

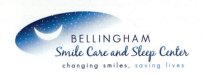

Good News for Treating Sleep Apnea without a CPAP Machine

Most people diagnosed with sleep apnea are told CPAP is their only treatment. That's just not true. Oral appliances are designated as first line treatment for mild to moderate sleep apnea and for anyone who can't adapt to or just can't tolerate their CPAP machine.

If you are diagnosed with sleep apnea, we can treat you with an easy to use, custom-fitted FDA approved dental appliance. These appliances can restore optimal, natural breathing—allowing you to get a healthy night's sleep. I use one myself for treating my sleep apnea. It has dramatically improved my health and stamina and I'm sleeping better than ever. Many people are not aware that a specially trained dentist can treat their sleep apnea.

Don't give up hope—there is an alternative. Successful obstructive sleep apnea treatment might just save your life—that's no exaggeration.

Why We Treat Sleep Apnea at The Bellingham Smile Care and Sleep Center

A number of years ago, I realized that I was getting very tired, especially while driving. I knew that was a key symptom of sleep apnea. In fact, Drowsy Driving kills more people on the road than drivers under the influence. I didn't think I was getting any less sleep than usual, but the driving issue caused me to get tested (an overnight sleep study). It turned out I had moderate sleep apnea, waking up about 17 times an hour because I would stop breathing. This was a literal wake-up call for me. I began researching what I could do through my dental practice to help myself and other people suffering with sleep apnea.

> "I had heard about alternatives to CPAP machines and in my online research I came across The Bellingham Care and Sleep Center. Right away I saw they had some alternatives for helping with the nightmare I called snoring.
>
> "I'd been dealing with snoring for a long time and it had caused some serious mental and physical issues for me. After reading what other patients had to say I decided to make the call and it was the best thing I ever did.
>
> "Dr. Prager talked to me about sleep apnea and he showed me an oral appliance he thought would work for me. I was so excited about not having to use a CPAP machine. After undergoing an overnight sleep test, I had the appliance made and I got the first good night of sleep I'd had in years—the very first time I slept with the appliance. And, I didn't snore! The appliance is amazing and I want to tell everyone if you have trouble with sleep apnea, snoring and sleeping, this device works!
>
> "I'm forever grateful to the team at The Bellingham Smile Care and Sleep Center. They gave me my life back."
>
> **Brandon Pappas – Bellingham, WA**

I discovered there were a number of dental sleep appliances that could treat sleep apnea, so after undergoing a rigorous program of specialized course work and education, I made myself one. I started sleeping better, I was less tired, and I was breathing better during the day. I proved it to myself—on myself! I personally did not want to wear a CPAP; in fact, the thought of wearing one caused me to resist getting tested for sleep apnea to begin with.

Once I had success with the appliance and knew it was a successful and comfortable treatment for sleep apnea, I pursued advanced certification in dental sleep medicine. I took dozens and dozens of hours of training in sleep apnea and related fields. I was determined to be the best trained dentist on sleep apnea in our corner of Northwestern Washington.

> "I came to Dr. Prager to explore a different treatment for sleep apnea because I couldn't transport my CPAP apparatus on a trip abroad. I had doubts, but Dr. Prager and his staff were very professional and polite. Each step of the oral appliance process was explained in detail. I have put aside my old CPAP equipment and now enjoy a trouble-free regimen of treatment using the oral appliance. I am extremely pleased with the entire experience and I am a firm believer in this type of treatment for sleep apnea. Thank you Dr. Prager!"
>
> John Euen – Bellingham, WA

Certification in dental sleep medicine requires fairly rigorous training, including significant course work, many hours of observation in a medical sleep lab, and written and practical exams. As of this printing I am the only dental member of all of the following academies practicing in Whatcom County: American Academy of Dental Sleep Medicine, Academy of Clinical Sleep Disorders Disciplines, and the American Academy of Sleep Medicine. I am honored to have earned Diplomate status with the Academy of Clinical Sleep Disorders Disciplines—the first dentist in the State of Washington to be so designated.

I feel that you have to have extensive education, training, and experience in the field of dental sleep medicine (which is not taught in dental school) in order to do the best for your patients. Studying dental sleep medicine has taught me a difficult lesson: there is something more important than teeth—which was tough for me to learn to accept—and that's breathing. If you can't breathe, it doesn't matter how nice your teeth are, or much else for that matter... More and more dentists are getting into treating snoring and/or sleep apnea. Some of them attend weekend courses offered by dental labs that specialize in a particular appliance. Some may not have any training, they just send an impression of patient's teeth to a dental lab, give the patient the appliance and tell them to go on the Internet and find out how to use it properly. The American Academy of Sleep Medicine and the American Academy of Dental Sleep Medicine have recommended that dentists only attempt treating obstructive sleep apnea after rigorous training.

I take a different approach than other dentists. First, I work with each patient to figure out what's going to work best for them. When it comes to solutions, one size does not fit all. I work with many different types of appliances and many different dental labs. Together, we'll find the solution that is best for you.

The bottom line is I know these appliances work—I wear one myself. I treated my own sleep apnea and I continue to wear my appliance every night and I'll wear it for the rest of my life. It's made a profound difference in the quality of my sleep, and as a result, in my energy level and quality of life.

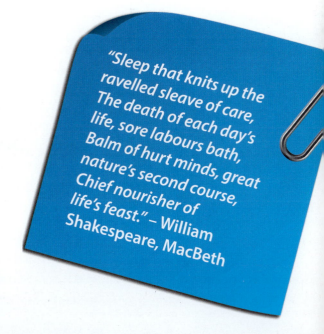

"Sleep that knits up the ravelled sleave of care, The death of each day's life, sore labours bath, Balm of hurt minds, great nature's second course, Chief nourisher of life's feast." – William Shakespeare, MacBeth

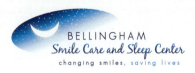
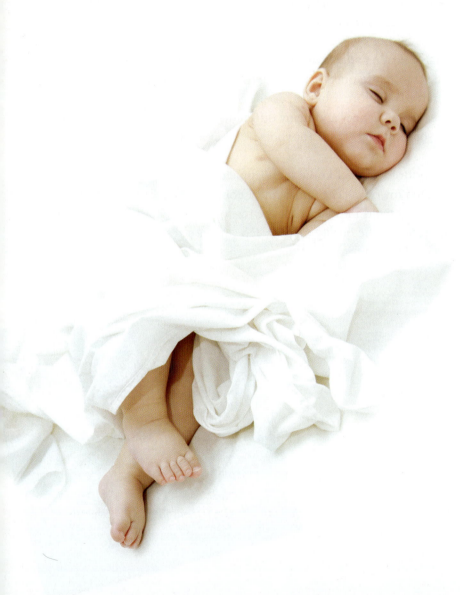

Chapter 17

Sleep Like a Baby, Wake Refreshed, Experience More Energy and Vitality

When it comes to breathing, we have a saying in dental sleep medicine: "The airway is King and the tongue is Queen." Dental appliances work by moving the lower jaw forward, which helps your tongue move forward which opens your throat and helps you to breathe. Your tongue is hooked into your jaw; if your jaw goes forward so does your tongue. And, the back of your tongue is huge; what we can see in the mirror is just the "tip of iceberg." When we lay back, the tongue can block our air flow. Humans are the only animal this is true of, because we've developed a throat anatomy that allows us to talk.

Correcting your breathing with a dental appliance can make a tremendous difference in the quality of your sleep and your life. When you sleep through the night and aren't waking up multiple times each hour, your body has time to do what it was designed to do: rest and replenish itself. Waking up rejuvenated, ready to take on the day can change everything—your outlook, your productivity, your overall health.

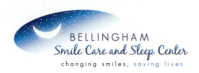

Very few dentists are qualified to provide what we offer in the area of sleep medicine. In fact, our sleep apnea treatment functions like a specialized medical practice inside our dental office. If you or someone you love might be suffering from sleep apnea—please, don't ignore it another minute—your life (or theirs) is at stake!

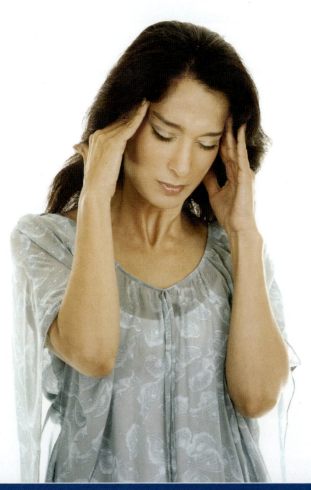

Chapter 18

Chronic Headaches and Migraines

"Really, you think a migraine is just a headache? And I suppose Godzilla is just a lizard."
– Author unknown

"Treated by a dentist? Really?" That's something we hear a lot around our office. Suffering from chronic headaches or migraines is flat-out miserable. There's just no other way to put it. I see patients whose lives are greatly diminished by headaches and pain they experience. It affects their relationships with family and friends—it can wreak havoc with their work and in many cases keeps them from enjoying leisure activities. They live in terror of the next episode. That's stressful, sad, and unnecessary.

- ☑ The National Headache Foundation has determined that over 45 million Americans suffer from headaches and migraines.

- ☑ The World Health Organization has noted that over 900,000 Americans experienced a migraine headache yesterday!

- ☑ The U.S. Agency for Healthcare Research and Quality has stated that over 3 million Americans went to a hospital emergency room seeking relief from headaches in 2010.

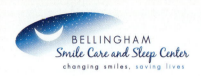

I know you probably don't associate dentists with treating headaches, but consider this. Your brain has an area we call the "headache center" located near the base of your skull. Right there is where all the nerves from the mouth, teeth, and jaw joints, and the muscles that move them intersect. The techno-medical term for this area is the trigeminal nerve center. Let's call it your TG nerve for now.

Your TG nerve is involved with your jaw, ligaments, and teeth and the muscle functions of your head and neck. If that nerve becomes unbalanced, your brain senses it, and guess what? Right. Headaches and pain are the result.

This TG nerve is in the area where we perform daily functions such as:

- Chewing
- Swallowing
- Breathing
- Eating
- Talking

All things we do every day, all day. And, if you have an imbalance in any of those vital functions, it has the potential to be aggravated thousands of times a day—literally! We open and close our mouths that many times each day. If you have a problem with any of those muscles, ligaments, or joints, it's like water torture—each individual drip isn't so bad, but non-stop, it will wreak havoc.

Your teeth aren't flat. Their surfaces look like small mountains and valleys. Yet, the muscles that move the jaw need to match up with the mountains and valleys like a lock and key when they come together. If they don't, you can be at risk for pain—just an annoyance or a raging headache or migraine that threatens to ruin your life.

"Before treatment with Dr. Prager I was having small but chronic headaches daily and at least one stronger headache each week. Every month I had one to two major migraines, even while taking prescription medication to prevent headaches. I was at the point that my life activities revolved around my headaches rather than family activities.

"As I come to the end of my treatment with Dr. Prager, I have been headache free for two weeks in a row and am no longer taking medication every day. This has been a life changing treatment and I would recommend it to anyone and everyone that suffers from headaches."

M Haug – Bellingham, WA

By the way, if you've ever felt that your headaches or migraines run your life, I want to say this to you: It's NOT your fault. So many people feel guilty or embarrassed, in part because anyone who doesn't suffer as you do can't really understand what you go through. Sure, they can be sympathetic, but at some point, it's tiring for them and they run out of patience. Yet, nothing has changed for you. We can all understand both sides, but it doesn't make it any easier. Not at all. And if you think you've tried EVERYTHING to defeat your headaches, just maybe you haven't . . .

"A migraine is like a tornado. It attacks fast, usually without warning, and wreaks havoc regardless of what's going on in your life at the moment." – Stephen Silberstein MD

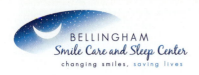

A Real and Lasting Solution to Headaches

Happily, I can say yes, there is! I know, you're thinking, but . . . you're a dentist, I don't get it. Believe me, I've heard that before. I'll let you in on a secret. Physicians mean well—they don't like to see their patients in pain. They want to provide relief. Their training is to treat headaches with drugs. Even if it does relieve the pain—and it doesn't always—it doesn't fix the underlying cause of the headaches, so they don't stop. Guess which medical professional works in the area where headaches occur? The dental physician. Medical doctors aren't aware of the advancements being made in dental medicine—why should they be? They have enough to keep up with in their own fields.

Not a lot of dentists have had special training in headaches, either. In fact, there are only 400 of us nationwide trained in the TruDenta system for dental headache treatments. The good news is we treat headaches without drugs or needles. In fact, our treatment is a "spa-like" dental therapy that is relaxing, soothing, feels great, and alleviates headaches in 93% of the patients we see. That's good news.

"I've suffered from headaches and migraines since college. That's more than 30 years of chronic headaches every single day, and migraines two to three times a week. I tried everything from acupuncture and herbal remedies to seeing a neurologist for many years. I have been prescribed many different drugs over time, and yet every morning I woke up with a headache.

"I went into Dr. Prager for dental work and he told me about his headache treatment program. They were really surprised to learn I had a headache every single day and they encouraged me to try treatment at their office.

"Honestly, I was really skeptical. I'd already tried so many things. I decided not to pursue it. Finally, my husband said to me, 'Why not try it? You have nothing to lose.' That made sense to me, so I decided to try it.

"Originally they thought maybe six to seven treatments would work. They had me keep progress notes, and while I wasn't cured after six treatments, I was having fewer headaches. I was getting better and better and after 12 treatments I wasn't waking up with headaches anymore and I wasn't having headaches during the day. The treatments were actually enjoyable, though at first I was very tender. Stassya (my dental neuro-muscular therapist) was very patient and kind and worked with me to find the best way to treat me since my face is so sensitive.

"I really thought I was going to have to live with chronic headaches and migraines the rest of my life. Now, I have an occasional headache if I forget to wear my night guard. Dr. Prager is very serious and focused and he's solved my problem for good!"

– Karen Yeung, Bellingham, WA

Did You Know?

The accumulated impact of just 600 anti-inflammatory pills like ibuprofen can cause permanent liver damage. That's just two pills a day for one year. Even if you don't take them every day, the cumulative effect is the same. You need a safe, natural, and lasting solution to relieve your pain and protect your precious organs.

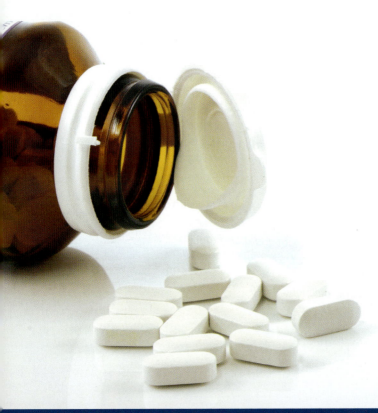

Chapter 19

Drugs Don't Cure Headaches

If you suffer from chronic headaches or migraines, you've probably got an assortment of pills handy—probably prescription and over-the-counter remedies. I know, sometimes they relieve the pain and sometimes they don't. There is one thing they do all the time and that is they accumulate in your system. Eventually that can harm your organs.

Scary Fact about Drugs

We are one of the most overmedicated countries in the world. We have more headaches, stress, and health problems than people in most other countries. We are sold on the idea of pills to relieve pain—aspirin, ibuprofen, acetaminophen, and other over-the-counter drugs as well as prescription drugs. And guess what? Side effects from prescription and non-prescription drugs are one of the top ten leading causes of death in this country.

That's alarming, don't you think? I do. Especially when there's an alternative. Since you're reading this book, you're fortunate to be within close distance to one of the few practices that might be able to help you solve your problem.

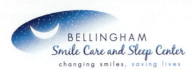
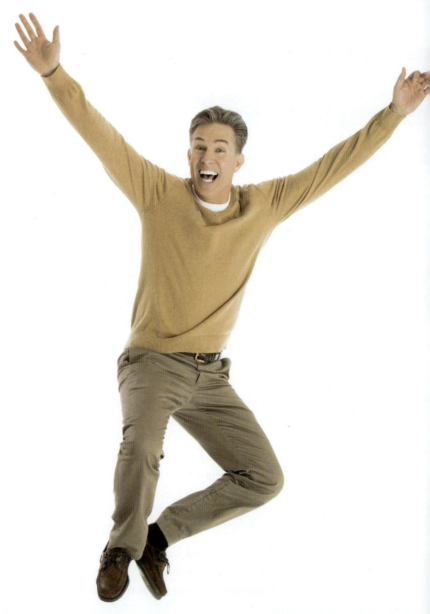

Chapter 20

Real and Lasting Headache Relief

Our office is among the one-half of one percent of the dental offices nationwide (that's right, 99.5% of practices don't offer this treatment) that have the TruDenta technology and training to diagnose the pain-causing dental force imbalances in your head and neck.

We can analyze your bite forces—in fact we're the only dental practice in our county that can—using the T-Scan Bite Force Analyzer. You've probably been to the dentist who checks to make sure you don't have any high or low spots—after a cavity has been filled, for example—by having you bite down on typewriter ribbon. They can see by the ink left on your teeth what needs adjusting.

What this method doesn't tell us is which teeth touch first and how much force they're exerting. Our T-Scan equipment analyzes your bite, including where, when, and how much force you're exerting. It's completely computerized and painless, so it's quick and easy, but it lets us identify—with pinpoint accuracy—exactly where the force imbalance is occurring.

Determining exactly where the dysfunction is, we know the source and strength of any force imbalance. This is important to understand as this muscle imbalance can contribute to 80% of headaches! Finding and correcting the imbalance can relieve jaw pain, headaches, and

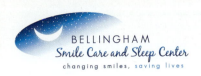

prevent (further) bone loss. Typically, a physician's treatment for headaches is to prescribe drugs. Drugs might mask the pain (and they don't always do that), but they don't cure the problem. Our approach allows us to diagnose the problem and rehabilitate the muscles, ligaments, and joints in the lower face that are responsible for headache pain.

Chapter 21

How Our Therapy Process Helps Your Headaches and Migraines

Your therapy is experienced in a relaxed, comfortable environment. We dim the lights and help you get comfortable. It's actually a pampering, soothing experience. I know, you may not associate the dentist's office with pampering and soothing—but you will!

Your therapist works on the muscles in your head, neck, and jaw, including your jaw joints. Muscles that have been chronically tense and in spasm relax as normal physiology is restored. Built-up waste products are released and proper blood flow is restored to your muscles and your "hot spots." We utilize therapeutic modalities such as ultrasound, micro-current, focused massage, and cold laser, on the areas of your head and neck that are triggers for headaches and migraines.

Part of your treatment regimen is focused home care—the restoration of your unbalanced muscles continues at home to gently bring you back into harmony, bringing an end to the relentless pain cycle you've been living with for too long.

Did You Know?

In our office, relieving your chronic headaches and migraines involves no needles, no pain, and no drugs of any kind. We combine sports medicine technology with advanced dental therapy. All done in a relaxing, spa-like, stress-free environment.

After Treatment, You Can Relieve Most Headaches on Your Own, at Home

To that end, we get you through the therapy process as quickly as possible and give you tools you can use at home, should you need them. If you ever feel a headache coming on, you can treat the headache yourself with a high degree of certainty you'll prevent the headache from happening or significantly decrease the intensity and frequency of the pain.

What is your headache and migraine pain costing you? Have you ever allowed yourself to think what your life could be like without your headaches and migraines?

If you suffer from headaches or migraines, you don't want to waste another precious moment of your life in pain. You can experience "normal" life again and do everything you've been missing. Patients who have received our treatment tell us their lives have improved in many ways:

- Less frequent, less intense, or no headaches or migraines
- Better, more restful sleep
- No more clenching or grinding of your teeth
- Reduced snoring
- No more sore facial and chewing muscles
- Reduced or no popping or clicking of their jaw joints

Please share this information with anyone you know who suffers from headaches. Knowing there's a possibility of living without pain and the compromised life that goes along with chronic pain, can be miraculous news for migraine and headache sufferers.

"I am so thankful for the opportunity to have received the specialized treatment for headaches and migraines. After the first treatment I no longer experienced the heavy and foggy head which I had on a daily basis.

"I have had a few headaches, but now have the tools to manage and get rid of them, which makes me feel in control and hopeful for the future. I can actually look forward to my future and have my quality of life back. My experience with you has been very positive and it's a wonderful place to be treated."

– Rose Klassen, British Columbia, Canada

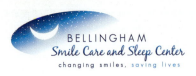
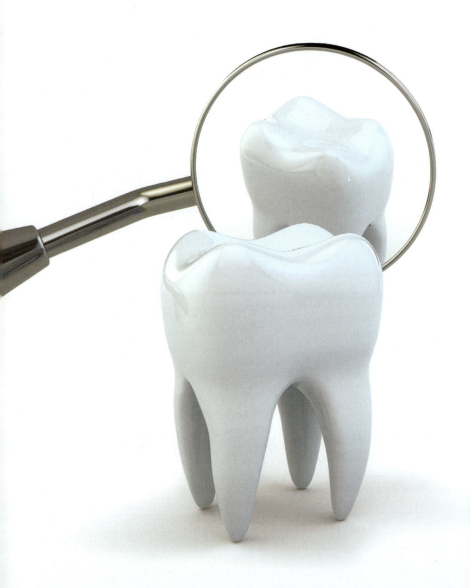

Chapter 22

Do You Offer "Regular Dental Services" like Cleaning, Filling Cavities, Crowns, and Preventive Work? You Bet!

I've gotten that question over the years from some new patients who are amazed at how unique our office is and think we might not do "regular garden variety dentistry" also . . . of course we do! You may have noticed—and I've experienced this myself visiting different doctors over the years—you aren't usually presented with options, you're told what to do as if it was the last word.

I like my patients to know what kinds of treatments and services are available to them at The Bellingham Smile Care and Sleep Center. It works with my philosophy of enhancing lives. I believe when you feel more in control of your experience, it works better for you. It's also less frightening when you understand your options.

BELLINGHAM
Smile Care and Sleep Center

"When I finally found the courage to go see Dr. Prager I had neglected my teeth for over 25 years. Many were broken or had fallen out altogether. There were several infections that were a threat to my overall health. I was embarrassed and ashamed of my mouth and did not want anyone poking around in what was a battlefield. When one of my front teeth broke I was trapped. I had to do something about it.

"I read about The Bellingham Smile Care and Sleep Center and thought it would be a comfortable place to be. I was more than correct in my assumption. I found the team to be totally non-judgmental and only interested in what was the best treatment for me. It gave me an overwhelming feeling of acceptance.

"My treatment included diagnosis, extraction, cavity filling, cleaning, and installation of a new smile. All this was done with the utmost professionalism and virtually no pain. There are no words to express how happy I am with my 'new look.'

"At The Bellingham Smile Care and Sleep Center, one is treated with caring and respect. There is a feeling of being surrounded by a loving family. Dr. Prager and the team he has assembled are wonderful and I can recommend them with my highest rating. I will look forward to my semi-annual visits."

Bob Currie – Bellingham, WA

Our High-Tech, State-of-the-Art "Regular" Dental Services

Low Dose Digital X-Rays
Digital X-rays use much less radiation—85% less, to be exact. X-ray technology is an important diagnostic tool—it can save lives. However, the less radiation you and your family are exposed to, the better. We help our patients every day with safer X-rays that many offices just don't offer.

Rotadent—a Kinder, Gentler Way to Brush
So much gum loss happens at our hand—literally. Ironically, it often happens to the most diligent brushers. We brush without thinking, and the most fastidious brushers scrub, scrub, and scrub some more. That's fine on the top of your tooth surfaces—they're enamel and tough. When you get to the sides of your teeth and use the same pressure, you can't help but brush your gums. Gums are fragile and as you brush them away you expose the dentin (the inside structure of your tooth)—making you more susceptible to developing cavities, tooth sensitivity, and loss of tooth structure.

I'd vote for taking manual toothbrushes out of everyone's hands. I'd have you use a Rotadent instead. Our patients have been using the gentle Rotadent with great results for more than 20 years. You don't need toothpaste with the Rotadent, which is a great thing, as toothpaste is incredibly abrasive and another cause of gum loss and gum recession. Not using toothpaste is radical . . . but we look at it differently. We have patients use an alcohol-free mouth rinse if they'd like the fresh clean taste that comes from brushing. Gentle, effective, and easy to use; we're trying to keep you from brushing away your gums and teeth—a very common problem we see today.

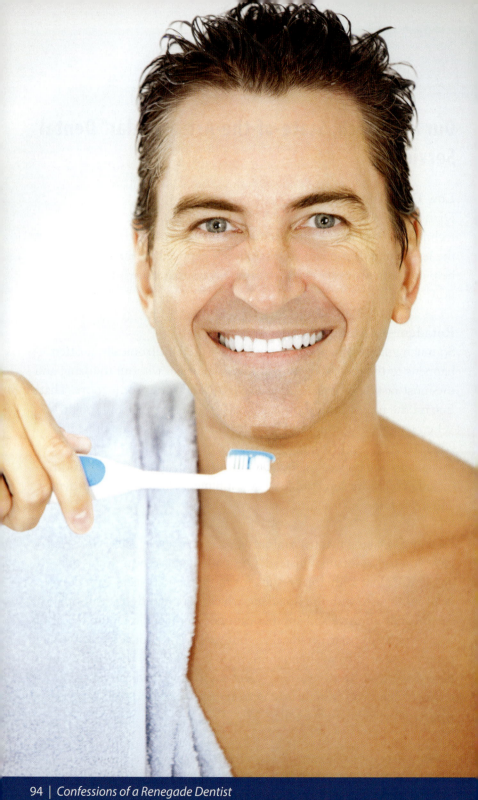

Chapter 23

Easy and Efficient Ways to Keep Your Teeth Clean, Even if You Hate Flossing

Hydro Floss

So many people absolutely hate to floss. So guess what they do? Avoid it altogether. Flossing gets what your toothbrush can't. There is a gentle, simple solution that's actually even more effective than the dreaded flossing.

Hydro Floss cleans between your teeth. It's a water jet that uses magnetized water, a fantastic alternative that our patients have been using successfully for more than ten years.

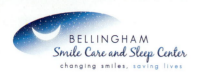
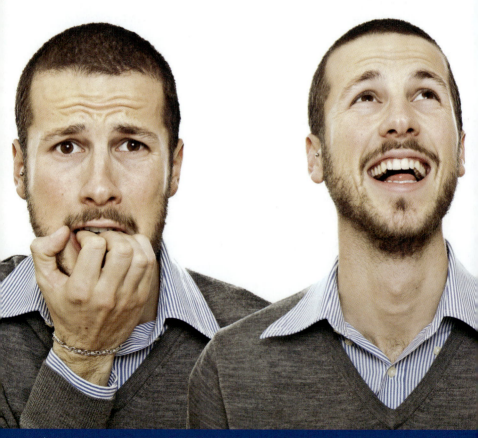

Chapter 24

I'm Terrified of the "Needle" and of Pain—Help!

The Wand
The Wand is a unique method of administering local anesthetic (numbing) that's way more patient friendly. You still get profoundly numb and it's way more comfortable than the traditional method. With the Wand I don't have to use the dreaded metal syringes to put your teeth to sleep while we pamper them. I have been using the Wand exclusively for more than fifteen years.

Tooth-Colored Composite Fillings— No Mercury Here
I haven't used mercury fillings since 1981! I was one of the first dentists in the United States to stop using mercury in patients' mouths. Composite fillings are strong and long lasting. They're tooth-colored, so you don't have that "mouth full of metal" look and they strengthen your teeth because they are bonded to your tooth structure.

Air Abrasion Tooth-Colored Fillings
In many cases, especially if a cavity is small, we can use Air Abrasion, a simple no shot/no drill method for filling small cavities.

Essentially the cavity is gently blown away with air and sterile sand

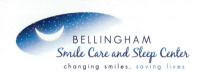

and we bond in a tooth-colored filling. These fillings are long lasting, comfortable, and cost less than regular fillings. Our office was the very first in Whatcom County to offer Air Abrasion Fillings. Our patients overwhelmingly prefer to have their fillings done with no shots and no drills. We've been using Air Abrasion fillings for twenty years. Yet, few dentists have incorporated this technology—less than 5% use it with their patients.

Crowns

Dental crowns strengthen and beautify teeth and we offer several different types.

All-porcelain crowns are the closest to the teeth Mother Nature gave you. Porcelain and gold crowns are an excellent combination of strength and beauty. Zirconia crowns are extremely strong and have the advantage of being tooth-colored. We use all-gold crowns when our overriding concern for a particular patient is strength and the need for longevity. We discuss all materials choices for crowns with our patients so they can choose the best crowns for their needs and desires.

Diagnodent

This technology is brilliant. It uses a painless laser to detect cavities long before they'd cause a problem. That means we can treat cavities with no shots and no drilling. You'll save money in the long run because we catch the problem while it's very simple to treat.

Oral Conscious Sedation

An oral sedative that relaxes you throughout the entire dental procedure. You have no memory of the procedure, which relieves anxiety and stress. This is a great solution for patients who could never sit through a dental appointment otherwise. We haven't had many requests to use this method since we started using NuCalm, which you read about earlier.

Root Canal

We know, root canal treatment is the butt of many jokes. However, when the only other option is extracting a tooth and losing it forever, root canal is an alternative that we'll use to save your natural tooth—always our first and foremost concern.

The Dental Button

This is a terrific anxiety-reducing device that puts you in complete control of the dental experience. You have a button that literally stops the procedure at any time for any reason. You simply press the button and everything stops so you are fully in charge. We are one of only two offices in Washington that uses this anxiety-reducing device.

> "The device used to stop the drill is amazing! It gives the patient control and a sense of security. I love this new innovation you have brought into your practice."
> – Judith Madjic
> Bellingham, WA

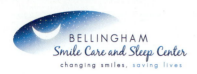
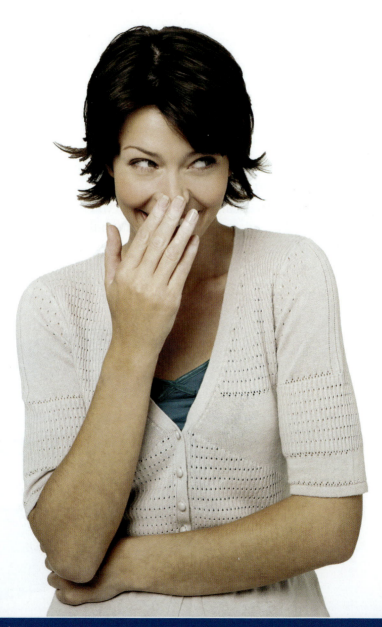

Chapter 25

I've Never Liked My Smile, What Can I Do?

I've been asked these kinds of questions by so many patients over the years:

- ☑ I've never liked my smile, is there anything you can do to help me?

- ☑ My teeth are crooked, can they be fixed?

- ☑ My teeth have gaps and I don't like the way they look, what can I do?

- ☑ I had braces as a teen, but now my teeth have all moved back; can they be re-aligned properly?

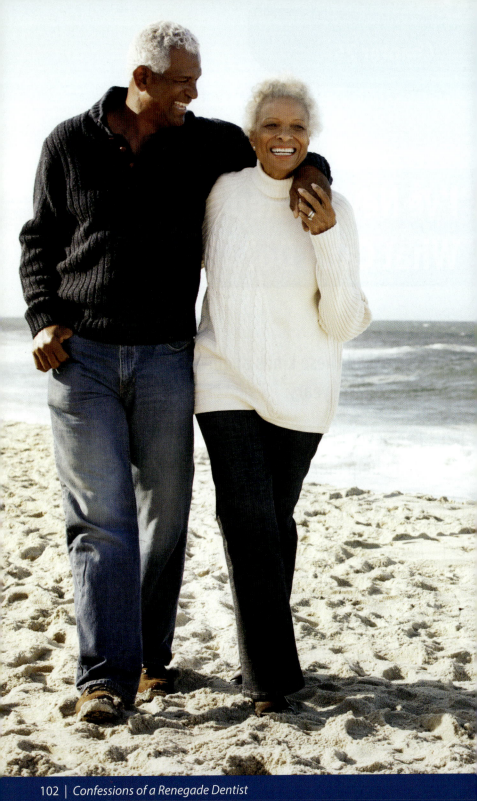

Cosmetic Dentistry Solutions Improve Your Smile, Enhance Your Looks, and Increase Your Confidence

> *"There is no weapon in the feminine armory to which men are so vulnerable as they are to a smile."* — Dorothy Dix

At The Bellingham Smile Care and Sleep Center, we offer a number of options to give you a beautiful smile you'll feel great about. Everything we do is for teens and adults who want an improved smile.

"I came to your office with hope for 'prettier teeth.' I didn't know what I wanted or what was available. I had met with other dentists but walked away from your office totally impressed with your thorough consultation and your attention to detail. I was also impressed with the whole spirit in your office—from the administrators on down.

"I so appreciated your commitment to details and excellence. My teeth look absolutely real and they have transformed my smile. Would it be too embarrassing to admit I smile at myself in the mirror a lot, just so I can see my new smile? You are truly an artist!"

Ginny Dye – Bellingham, WA

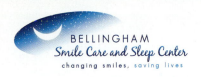

Cosmetic Orthodontic Options

We have three methods we use and they all focus on the teeth that show when you smile. These are not procedures intended to make major changes to your bite.

Fastbraces®
Fastbraces® is an orthodontic technique perfected over 20 years by an orthodontist in Texas. It allows us to safely straighten your teeth using either clear or metal braces in as little as 3 months to about a year—shorter than conventional braces treatment time and more affordable. We are the only office in our area providing Fastbraces® treatment for teens and adults.

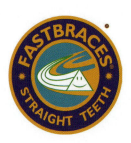

Inman Aligner
The Inman Aligner is a removable appliance you wear for 18-20 hours a day that straightens your front teeth quickly and safely. It is the fastest and most affordable option we offer to straighten your teeth. Invented in England, we are the first dental office to bring it to our corner of Northwestern Washington.

Clear Correct
Like Invisalign, this treatment uses clear retainers to gently move your teeth into the desired position. You remove the aligners to eat and brush. This treatment takes longer than the other 2 highlighted here, but if you want your entire orthodontic treatment to be nearly invisible, then Clear Correct is for you.

Breakthrough Cosmetic Restorative Dentistry and Smile Redesign Services

We take special care with our smile redesign service and go the extra mile so you can "test" your smile before it becomes permanent. We recreate your new smile in wax first—before we touch your teeth—so you can see if you love the look. You can take it home, get opinions from the people who care about you, and get a sense of what your new smile will look like. We also do custom computer imaging so you can see a picture of what your new smile will look like and we can make adjustments so you get exactly what you want. From there, we'll proceed to use one of two techniques:

Porcelain Veneers
Allow us to give you the smile of your dreams by changing the shape, crookedness, color, and spacing of your teeth in just two visits.

DuraThin Veneers
We use super-thin, yet ultra-strong porcelain to change your smile from dull to dazzling in the most comfortable way possible. In many instances, no shots are required. DuraThin veneers don't require much smoothing of your tooth, so they don't compromise the tooth structure itself.

"Little did I know I'd find the finest dentist on the planet through a Google search. Years of nightly tooth grinding has worn my teeth down to nubs, so I was in search of a dentist who could restore my teeth.

"I also wanted a dentist who could provide me with comfortable care, as when I was a child I had the displeasure of having some cavities filled by a dentist who skimped on Novocain, and I've been nervous about dentists in general ever since...

continued on the next page

..."Dr. Prager was fabulous. He took as much time as needed to answer all my questions in a patient manner and did not rush anything I was unsure about. He explained the veneer process from beginning to end, and I sensed he was meticulous in his work.

"During the veneer process, I further marveled at just how meticulous he really was. Every part of the process was done in a step-by-step careful manner. If something wasn't just right, it was done again until he achieved perfection.

"I am thrilled with the outcome and my new smile. The end result was far above my expectations, and I cannot thank Dr. Prager and his staff enough for a job well done."

Monica Erickson - Bellingham, WA

Expert's Choice Tooth Whitening
If you're after a gleaming smile, you're in the right place. Some of our patients complained about sensitivity with some of the whitening treatments they'd used in the past. We searched out the best in-office zero-sensitivity tooth whitener there is and that's what we use exclusively. We are the only office in Whatcom and Skagit Counties using Expert's Choice in-office teeth whitening. The procedure is quick—it takes only 20 minutes—and it's way less expensive than other treatments you may have had in the past. Affordable, effective, zero-sensitivity teeth whitening exists, and you'll find it here!

"I told my dentist my teeth were going yellow. He told me to wear a brown tie." – Rodney Dangerfield

Chapter 26

FACE IT—TFE is the Best Way to Show Off Your Smile

What the heck is TFE you ask? TFE stands for Total Facial Esthetics. Your face frames your smile and if you think about it, a youthful smile in an older-looking face creates disharmony.

What can we do to help? Botox and Dermal Fillers. Botox allows us to smooth out lines and wrinkles around your lips, brow, forehead, eyes and more to give your face a relaxed and youthful look. Dermal fillers allow us to actually "fill-in" lines and folds around your face taking years off almost instantly. Botox and Dermal fillers combined show off your youthful smile in the best way possible—it's the "Total Package."

Very few dentists are trained in TFE. We are one of the very few offices in our area that provide TFE.

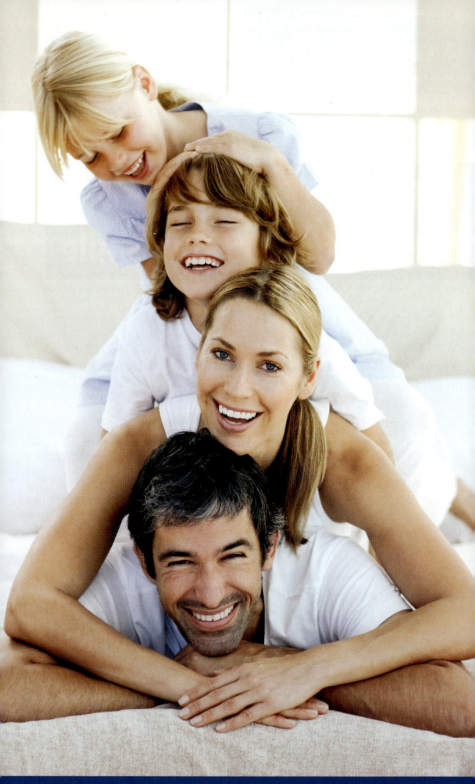

Chapter 27

Free "Teeth Whitening for Life"

We have a great program at The Bellingham Smile Care and Sleep Center. If you enroll in our free "Teeth Whitening for Life" program, we'll whiten your teeth for free—

FOREVER

—as long as you keep your dental maintenance appointments and keep your mouth healthy. After your cleaning visits we give you special teeth whitening gel to use between visits to keep your smile white and bright. You'll love this program.

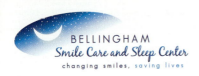
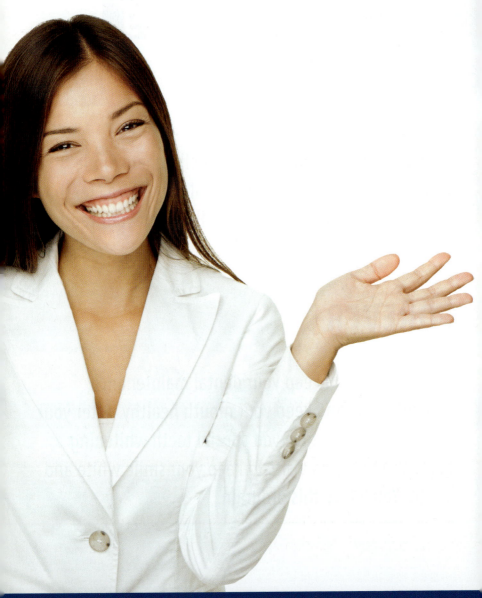

Chapter 28

Last Word

Thanks for taking this journey with me. Dental technology and the remarkable help we can give our patients have changed radically, particularly in the last 25 years. I've committed to helping my patients find solutions that are safe, comfortable, reliable, and in many cases enable me to save their natural teeth. Our health is a precious asset. You can lose any material possession, you can lose your job, even your home or a relationship, and though those experiences might be painful and take time to recover from, they're all replaceable—eventually. Not so with your health. You must care for your health and protect it carefully; once it's lost, you can't always get it back. And without your health, the quality of your life can change dramatically.

So much can be done today with prevention and forethought and taking the time to seek out the treatments—and the health care professionals—who are a fit for you and who you can trust to give you the best care.

If you're looking for a caring, compassionate dental practice—a place that is actually a pleasure to visit and where you know that everyone has your best interests at heart and the most current technology and methods using the least invasive procedures possible, then please call us or stop by for a visit. We'll make you feel welcome and if you're like a lot of our patients, you'll be relieved that you've found a place for superior care where we'll make sure you're relaxed and comfortable—and equally important, heard and listened to.

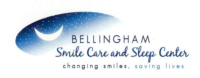

Schedule a complimentary consult and get to know us a bit, see if we'd be a fit for your needs. We know you might not be in the habit of "shopping around" for health services, but we have a new approach. That approach is about you finding something that works and works well for your needs.

We encourage you to talk to us and see if we can be that resource for you. We do things differently at The Bellingham Smile Care and Sleep Center and we make what is so often a dreaded visit to the dentist comfortable—some patients even tells us it's a pleasure . . . imagine! The added benefit? Great health and no more guilt about not doing what you know is in your best interest.

> "Dr. Prager, you are the most comforting physician I have ever experienced. Your office is modern with new technical equipment. Your staff greets each person and provides a very comforting reception and seldom is there any waiting. You, your staff, and your entire office create a very uplifting, accomplished, and calming environment to reassure hesitant customers that their experience is going to be okay. Once one has had an experience in Dr. Prager's care they lose all their apprehension towards 'Going to the Dentist,' because it truly is a painless and pleasant experience. While having your teeth cleaned by an excellent hygienist, you can watch a fascinating documentary on a TV screen. Dr. Prager talks to each patient and assures them of his team's capabilities to accomplish your dental needs. Dr. Prager has transformed an uncomfortable but necessary distressing business into a pleasing and peaceful professional practice that encompasses dentistry and many other aspects of properly caring and feeling good about ourselves. Thank you for all your dedicated work."
>
> John Greene – Anacortes, WA

Finally, if you have questions about anything you've read—reach out—we're accessible and easy to reach. I hope to have the opportunity to meet you and perhaps contribute to improving your health increasing your confidence and enhancing the quality of your life.

Dr. Jeffrey R. Prager
The Bellingham Smile Care and Sleep Center
1420 King Street, Suite B
Bellingham, WA 98229
360-671-4552
info@bellinghamsmiles.com
www.bellinghamsmiles.com

Learn more about
The Bellingham Smile Care and Sleep Center

About Dr. Jeffrey R. Prager

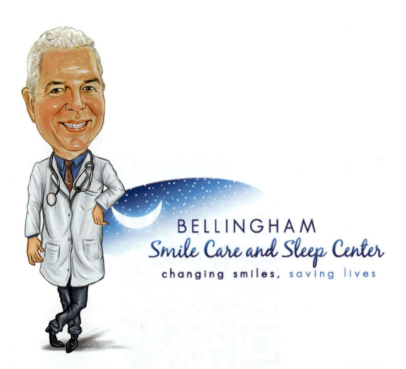

Jeffrey R. Prager DDS, D.ACSDD is a Baby-Boomer born in San Diego who has spent just about his entire life traveling up the West Coast—you might call him "Mono-Coastal."

After graduating from high school in San Diego, he moved up the coast to West Los Angeles where he attended UCLA. Jeffrey spent his senior year as an exchange student at the University of Sussex in England. He graduated Phi Beta Kappa, Summa Cum Laude from UCLA with a bachelor's degree in Zoology. He was accepted into the UCLA School of Dentistry as a Regent's Scholar and graduated in 1978 with his Doctor of Dental Surgery degree and went on to complete his General Practice Residency at the Wadsworth/Brentwood VA Medical Center in West Los Angeles.

Continuing his northward journey up the coast, he was appointed Staff Dentist at the Seattle VA Medical Center Dental Clinic where he practiced for three years before entering private dental practice as an associate in the Seattle area.

Another move up the coast took him to Bellingham in 1985 where he opened his own practice in March of 1987. Dr. Prager has practiced in Bellingham for over 28 years and has helped thousands of his patients improve their health, increase their confidence, and enhance the quality of their lives—that remains his focus, passion, and dedication to this day.

Dr. Prager is a member of the American Dental Association, The Washington State Dental Association, The Mount Baker District Dental Society, The International Academy of Oral Medicine and Toxicology, The Institute of Advanced Laser Dentistry, American Academy of Cosmetic Dentistry, American Academy of Facial Esthetics, The American Academy of Sleep Medicine, Dental Organization for Conscious Sedation, The American Academy of Dental Sleep Medicine, and the Academy of Clinical Sleep Disorders Disciplines where he serves as Director of United States Regions.